D1628335

Royal National

disorders of | a guide for

vision in | teachers and

children | carers

Richard Bowman

Ruth Bowman

Gordon Dutton

RNIB

Richard JC Bowman, *MA FRCOphth, Specialist Registrar in Ophthalmology, Great Ormond Street Hospital for Children, London*

Ruth F Bowman, *MA PGCE, Adv Dip in Ed Studies for Children with Disabilities of Sight, Teacher in Charge, Visual Impairment Unit, Jubilee Primary School, London*

Gordon N Dutton, *MD FRCOphth, Professor of Visual Science, Caledonian University and Consultant Ophthalmologist, Royal Hospital for Sick Children, Glasgow*

Further copies of this book can be purchased from RNIB Book Sales Service, c/o RNIB Customer Services Centre, PO Box 173, Peterborough PE2 6WS
Tel: 0845 7023153 Fax: 01733 371555 Email: cservices@rnib.org.uk

First published August 2001
by RNIB, 224 Great Portland Street, London W1W 5AA
© RNIB 2001

Printed and bound by Briden Print Ltd

The views in this book are those of the authors and may not be those of RNIB or the establishments listed above.

ISBN 1 85878 213 9

CONTENTS

WITHDRAWN

List of figures and plates   5
Introduction   8

CHAPTER 1 - *WHAT IS VISION AND HOW DO WE SEE?*   9

- The eye   9
- The seeing nerves   16
- The seeing brain   17

CHAPTER 2 - *ASSESSMENT AND MEASUREMENT OF VISION*   29

- History taking   30
- Refraction   33
- Refractive errors   35
- Visual acuity   38
- Functional acuity   42
- Visual fields   45
- Contrast sensitivity   51
- Electrical tests of vision   51
- Colour vision and colour contrast   53

CHAPTER 3 - *DISORDERS OF THE VISUAL SYSTEM AND THEIR IMPLICATIONS*   55

- The front of the eye   55
- The whole eye   66
- The back of the eye   86
- The seeing nerves   104
- The seeing brain   107

•	Motivation for learning	120
•	Creating an optimum environment	123
•	Materials which aid functional vision	126
•	Training in the use of functional vision	137

Appendix A - Glossary of terms	146
Appendix B - Blindness and visual impairment definitions	157
Appendix C - Common myths	159
Bibliography	161
Recommended reading	162
Index	163

LIST OF FIGURES

Figures	Description	Page
Fig 1.1	Diagram of the eyeball	10
Fig 1.2	Accommodation	11
Fig 1.3	Converting light	13
Fig 1.4	Normal focus	15
Fig 1.5a	The visual pathways from the eyes to the back of the brain	18
Fig 1.5b	Side on view of visual pathways	19
Fig 1.6	Specialised areas of the brain	25
Fig 1.7	Diagram showing the probable nervous pathways involved in reading a sentence and repeating it aloud	27
Fig 2.1	Normal sight, short sight, long sight	34
Fig 2.2	The closer an object is to the eye, the larger it appears	36
Fig 2.3a	Distance visual acuity: Snellen Charts	38
Fig 2.3b	Distance visual acuity: Snellen Charts	40
Fig 2.4	Near visual acuity: Maclure test	44
Fig 2.5a	Visual path of each eye is cut off by the nose	46
Fig 2.5b	3D map visual field of right eye	47
Fig 2.6	The normal blind spot	48
Fig 4.1	Size of print and font	127
Fig 4.2	Different point sizes	127

LIST OF PLATES

Plate	Description	Page
Plate 1	Cosmetically noticeable and visual impairing corneal scars of both eyes caused by Vitamin A deficiency. *(Photograph acknowledgement: Clare Gilbert, International Centre for Eye Health, London)*	78
Plate 2	Fundus	78
Plate 3	Colour confusion	78
Plate 4	Cardiff acuity cards	78
Plate 5	View with a visual acuity of 6/18	78
Plate 6	Blurred focus due to uncorrected refractive error	79
Plate 7	Reduced visual acuity (3/60)	79
Plate 8	Possible effect of nystagmus on vision	79
Plate 9	Topcon perimeter	79
Plate 10	Confrontational visual field testing	79
Plate 11	Worksheet: Normal visual field	80
Plate 12	Worksheet: Peripheral visual field loss	80
Plate 13	Hall: Normal visual field	80
Plate 14	Hall: Central visual field loss	80
Plate 15	Left sided visual loss (homonymous hemianopia)	80
Plate 16	Interrupted visual field	81
Plate 17	Contrast sensitivity test	81
Plate 18	Electroretinography (ERG) testing using skin electrodes *(Photograph acknowledgement: Michael Bradnam, Dept of Electrophysiology, RHSC, Glasgow)*	81

LIST OF PLATES continued.....

Plate	Description	Page
Plate 19	Ishihara test	81
Plate 20	Pastel coloured chips to be arranged by child as developed by Lea Hyvarinen	81
Plate 21	Congenital abnormality of the cornea	82
Plate 22	Keratoconus	82
Plate 23	Cataract	82
Plate 24	Aphakic spectacles	82
Plate 25	Coloboma	82
Plate 26	Albinism	83
Plate 27	Photophobia	83
Plate 28	Aniridia	83
Plate 29	Childhood glaucoma (buphthalmos)	83
Plate 30	Retinoblastoma	83
Plate 31	Retinitis pigmentosa	84
Plate 32	Hand-held LVAs	84
Plate 33	x8 illuminated LVA	84
Plate 34	Magnification of maps	84
Plate 35	Stand magnifiers	84
Plate 36	Spectacle mounted magnifier	85
Plate 37	Telescopic systems	85
Plate 38	Closed circuit TVs (CCTVs)	85

INTRODUCTION

This book describes the many different types of visual impairment and how they affect children's vision in different circumstances. It suggests ways of adapting educational strategies, resources and the learning environment to enable children with impaired vision to reach their full educational potential.

The first chapter explains how each part of the eye works and how different parts of the brain are responsible for particular aspects of what we see. The second chapter explains the various ways of assessing and measuring what a child can see. Chapter 3 deals with individual conditions and diseases that lead to visual impairment and considers educational implications for each. The final chapter looks in more detail at specific educational strategies for children with visual impairment and is followed by a comprehensive glossary of terms. In addition to illustrations alongside the text, colour photographs showing eye conditions and low vision aids appear in the centre of the book.

There are many causes of poor sight, each with its own peculiarities, which impair vision in different ways. For example, conditions that let too much light into the eye result in a significant reduction of vision in bright sunlight. Poorly developed optic nerves can cause vision which is a bit like looking through a colander. Brain damage can result in loss of half the vision to one side and in some children can seriously impair their ability to 'see' and understand complex pictorial material.

Assessment of functional vision needs to be carried out on a regular formal basis. In addition a day to day intuitive assessment of what the child is seeing and not seeing is a pre-requisite for planning an ongoing optimal educational strategy.

Armed with an understanding of the visual impairment, the central task for teachers is to devise teaching and learning strategies which circumvent any barriers to accessing knowledge and information. The aim is to ensure that children are not educationally disadvantaged on account of poor vision.

For ease of reading, we have alternated the use of he and she when referring to a child.

CHAPTER 1

WHAT IS VISION AND HOW DO WE SEE?

The fact that 40% of the human brain is devoted to processing visual information shows the complexity and importance of this remarkable sense. Such complexity means that vision is vulnerable to a wide variety of disorders giving rise to a wide range of different effects with many different implications for the child and his or her education. A basic understanding of the structures involved in seeing, from the eye through to the brain is therefore essential to understanding and dealing with the range of problems which children with various visual impairments may experience.

THE EYE

The cornea
A diagram of the eye is shown in **Figure 1.1**. The front surface of the eye, the cornea, is a transparent, smoothly curved surface for focusing light into the eye (the cornea provides most of the eye's focusing power). The surface is kept smooth and in good condition by tears which are spread over the surface by normal blinking. Loss of transparency due to scarring is a common cause of visual impairment in children in developing countries (often being related to measles and malnutrition, **Plate 1**) but is rare in more affluent countries. A scarred or white cornea can also cause a cosmetic problem for the child. The cornea is continuous with the white of the eye or sclera which makes up the rest of the external wall of the eye **(see Figure 1.1)**.

The lens
The rest of the eye's focusing power is provided by the lens inside the eye which is also transparent and contributes the variable focus necessary for the eye to be able to see objects both in the distance and close up. This variability is possible because the lens is elastic and is suspended from the ciliary muscle by ligaments or zonules.

Contraction of this muscle allows the lens to become a thicker and rounder shape with the stronger focusing power necessary for seeing near objects. This process is known as accommodation **(Figure 1.2)**. Loss of transparency in the lens can be due to a wide variety of causes and is called cataract. Although it is much more common in older people, it is also a major cause of visual impairment in children worldwide.

FIGURE 1.1 - *Diagram of the eyeball from above*

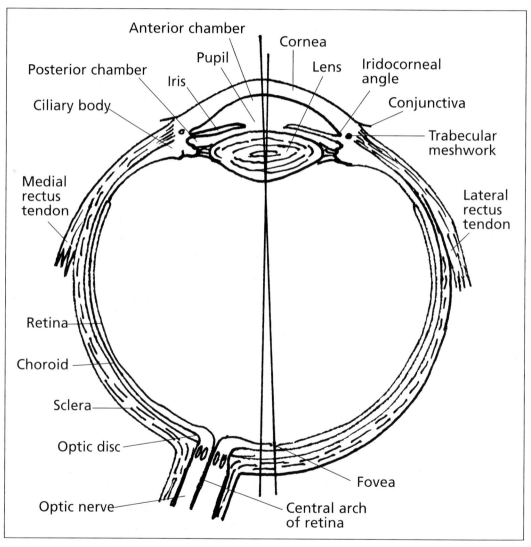

FIGURE 1.2 - *Accommodation. The solid lines represent the shape of the lens, iris, and ciliary body at rest, and the dotted lines represent the shape during accommodation.*

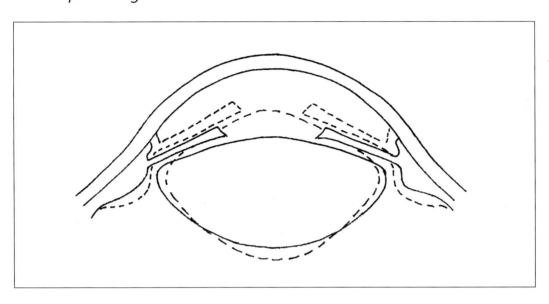

The fluid of the eye

Figure 1.1 shows that between the cornea and the lens is the anterior chamber which is filled with a transparent watery fluid, aqueous humour. This is continually pumped into the eye by the ciliary body and is continually drained out through a channel in the cleft (or angle) between the cornea and iris. The function of the aqueous humour is to provide oxygen and nutrients to the inside of the cornea and to the lens. In most other parts of the body this function is performed by blood but blood is red and the requirement for transparency of the eye has led to the production of this alternative to blood. The balance between the inflow and outflow of aqueous humour is responsible for the pressure of the eye. If the ciliary body fails to produce aqueous humour, the eye has no pressure and collapses, losing its shape (phthisis); if the outflow is blocked then the pressure inside the eye rises, which can cause glaucoma. This can damage vision and in children (whose sclerae are more elastic than adults') can cause enlargement of the eye known as 'buphthalmos' (from the ancient Greek meaning 'the eye of an ox').

The iris and pupil

The iris is the thin layer of muscle situated just in front of the lens and is the visible coloured part of the eye. It contains a central opening, the pupil, which varies in size according to the light level. In dim light the pupil gets bigger to maximise the amount of light entering the eye and in bright conditions it gets smaller to limit light entry. The main function of the pupil however, is to allow some degree of simultaneous focusing on targets at different distances away, in a similar way that reducing the aperture of a camera allows both the foreground and the background of a photograph to appear in focus. There are some conditions in which the iris is either absent (aniridia) or lacking pigment (albinism) and this control mechanism is therefore deficient.

Between the lens and the retina lies a transparent gel, the vitreous, occupying two thirds of the volume of the eye. Its transparency allows focused light to pass through to the retina.

The retina

The function of all the structures outlined above is to produce a clear and focused image on the retina, which is the 'screen' of the eye, and is analogous to the film in a camera (see Chapter 2 for more details of this optical arrangement). **Plate 2** illustrates the view of the retina seen by an ophthalmologist or optometrist looking into the eye with an ophthalmoscope (the instrument used to examine the retina, consisting of a torch and lens combination). The major landmarks are the optic disc which is the exit of the optic nerve which will be described later, and the macula which is the area about 4mm across and which includes the fovea (the most important point in the retina for detailed central vision) at its centre.

The retina is divided into two layers, the inner 'nerve' or neural layer and the outer pigment layer. The neural retina contains the cells (called rods and cones, or photoreceptors) which convert light into electrical signals which are eventually interpreted by the brain as a visual image **(Figure 1.3)**. This process depends on the presence in the rods and cones of substances (called photopigments) which change

FIGURE 1.3 - *Converting light*

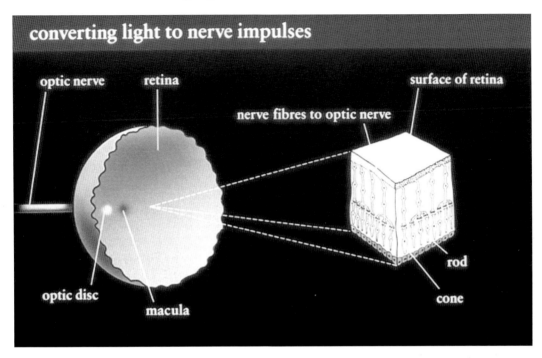

converting light to nerve impulses

optic nerve   retina   surface of retina

nerve fibres to optic nerve

rod

optic disc   cone

macula

the shape of their molecules when they absorb light energy. (These substances consist of a protein molecule linked to another molecule closely related to vitamin A (retinene).) The shape change in these molecules results in an electrical signal being sent to the optic nerve and then to the brain for interpretation. Thus there is a conversion of energy forms from the light coming into the eye, through chemical changes in the receptors, to electrical signals generated in the nerve fibres to the brain.

There are two different types of photoreceptor in the retina, rods and cones. It is important to appreciate the difference between rods and cones not only because they are responsible for quite different aspects of vision but also because some of the commonest causes of visual impairment (eg retinitis pigmentosa and cone dystrophies) may predominantly affect either the rods or the cones with very different visual implications for the child.

The rods are mainly responsible for vision in dim light and produce images consisting of varying shades of black and white, while the cones work in bright light, detect fine detail and are responsible for colour vision. The density of the rods and cones varies in different parts of the retina. The rods are absent at the fovea, the area about 2mm across responsible for discerning fine detail **(Plate 2)**. The cones on the other hand are most dense at the fovea. Both rods and cones contain photopigments (light-sensitive molecules), but whereas rods all contain the same photopigment, the cones are of three different types, each type containing a different photopigment. One group of cones responds especially to blue light, one group to red and one to green light. Hence the rods cannot respond to colour (we can't see colours in the dark) but the cones do.

Light and dark adaptation:
The eye has the ability to respond to a remarkably large range of different brightnesses. If you spend a considerable time in brightly coloured surroundings and then move to a dimly lit environment, the retinas become slowly more sensitive to dim light as you become accustomed to the dark. This is called dark adaptation and is nearly complete in about twenty minutes. On the other hand when you pass suddenly from a dim to a brightly lit environment, the light seems intensely and even uncomfortably bright until the eyes adapt to the increased illumination. This adaptation occurs over about five minutes and is called light adaptation. The cones and rods undergo dark adaptation separately, the cones adapting more quickly to the dark, but to a lesser degree than the rods which are more important for night vision.

Central and peripheral vision:
If a straight line is drawn between the object being looked at and the eye, through the centre of its cornea, it would hit the retina at the fovea. It is the fovea where the image of the object being looked at directly is focused **(Figure 1.4)**. Other objects at increasing distances to the side of the object being looked at are focused onto other areas of the retina at increasing distances from the fovea. This means that the part of the retina with the greatest resolving power for fine detail

FIGURE 1.4 - *Normal focus*

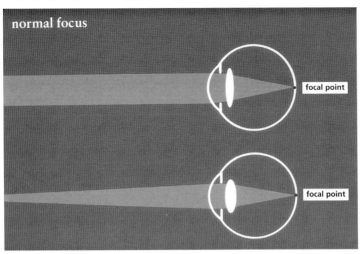

(the fovea) is directed at the object of interest or fixation point. The maximum resolving power of the eye (ie the finest detail which can be seen) is an important measurement of visual function and is termed visual acuity. Visual acuity is the most frequently recorded measurement of visual function since the ability to make out or resolve fine detail concerning the object of regard is essential to many of the visual tasks that we perform, particularly in the school environment, such as reading and writing. If you imagine looking at a single object in the middle of a room, there is a visual impression of the rest of the room, though it is not seen in fine detail. This is called our 'peripheral field', or 'field of vision' and is received by the receptors outside the macula. It is very important to our perception of the world around us and enables us to navigate through it. This peripheral vision can be measured by mapping out what is called the visual field, which simply means the total area that can be seen by one or both eyes in any particular position. The outer visual field is very sensitive to movement. When you move through a crowded environment you don't bump into things, even though you do not look directly at them. Similarly, when you run up a flight of stairs you don't usually look at each step directly. The visual field gives us remarkable sensitivity to movement which accounts for the tremendous mobility that some children have despite profound loss of central vision. (When a child is moving through a room, stationary objects are moving in visual terms.) More detailed explanations and implications of the terms visual acuity and visual field, together with some details of their measurement are given in Chapter 2. The outer or pigment layer of the retina consists of a single layer of cells with numerous functions including the absorption of stray light, and the formation (from vitamin A) of the photopigments needed by the rods and cones.

Between the pigment layer of the retina and the sclera is the 'choroid'. This is another pigmented layer which is well supplied with blood vessels (unlike many other parts of the eye which need to be transparent) and which is joined to the iris and ciliary body, all three together being termed the 'uvea' **(see Figure 1.1)**. Its main function is the nourishment of parts of the eye, especially the retina. The retinal blood vessels shown in **Plate 2** only nourish the inner part of the retina; the rest is supplied by the choroid. If the retina becomes separated from the choroid, as happens in retinal detachment, then it can suffer permanent damage due to oxygen starvation (similar to the brain damage which results from a stroke). If the macula becomes detached, the central vision will be affected, but if the detachment does not involve the macula, then only an area of peripheral vision, corresponding to the area of detached retina, will be impaired.

THE SEEING NERVES

Electrical signals from the rods and cones are transmitted through other cells in the neural retina to the ganglion cells. These are nerve cells with long fibres which pass from the cell through the optic disc (where all the fibres converge from the other ganglion cells from different positions throughout the retina) and into the brain. Together these fibres form the optic nerve which leaves the eye at the optic disc **(see Plate 2)**. All visual information from the retina leaves the eye through the optic nerve and hence the optic disc is a very important structure. Approximately 1.2 million nerve fibres are found in each optic nerve and when the two eyes are taken in combination this is estimated to contribute about 40% of all input to the brain! Unfortunately the nerves are susceptible to damage from many causes, for example, raised intra-ocular pressure, which can cause permanent visual field loss. This combination of damage is called glaucoma **(see p11)**.

The crossover

The route taken by the visual signal once it leaves each eye on its way to the visual parts of the brain is shown in **Figure 1.5a.** The optic nerve passes back to the brain through the bony cavity in the skull which encloses the eyeball (the orbit). In the skull it meets the optic nerve from the other eye at what is called the optic chiasm or crossover point. From there the visual message is transmitted further into the brain by connecting pathways called optic tracts. In general the right side of the brain responds to and controls things on the left side of the body whereas the left side of the brain correspondingly responds to and controls things on the right side of the body (thus a stroke affecting the right side of the brain may cause a left sided paralysis). This organisation of the brain applies to vision as well so that although each eye sees objects in both sides of the visual field, at the crossover all the information from the right side of the visual field (from both eyes) is passed to the left side of the brain and all information from the left side of the visual field (from both eyes) is passed to the right side of the brain **(see Figure 1.5a)**. Thus the crossover is very important when considering visual impairment because any damage to the left eye or optic nerve still leaves a full visual field from the right eye (which you can simulate by closing the left eye) but any damage to the left side of the pathway behind the chiasm may interfere with all vision from the right side of the visual field of each eye (a right hemianopia, meaning half blind on the right side) and likewise any damage to the right side of the pathway behind the chiasm may produce a left hemianopia **(see Plate 15)**.

THE SEEING BRAIN

From the chiasm the visual signal travels in nerve bundles (called optic tracts) to the back of the brain to a region called the visual cortex. The cortex consists of the surface layers of the brain and is the site of what is called higher brain function (eg conscious visual perceptions, or deliberate decision making). The size of the cortex is much bigger than in most animal brains, corresponding to the advanced intellectual function of humans. It is the cortex where the visual signals are

FIGURE 1.5a - *The visual pathways from the eyes to the back of the brain*

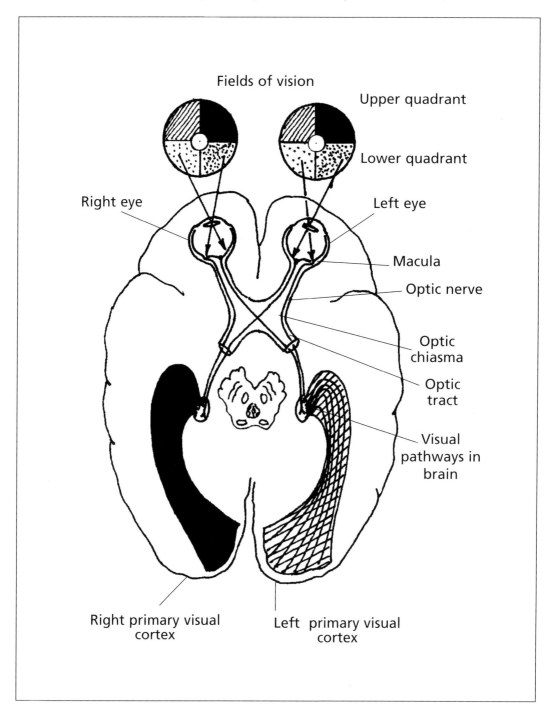

FIGURE 1.5b - *Side on view of visual pathways*

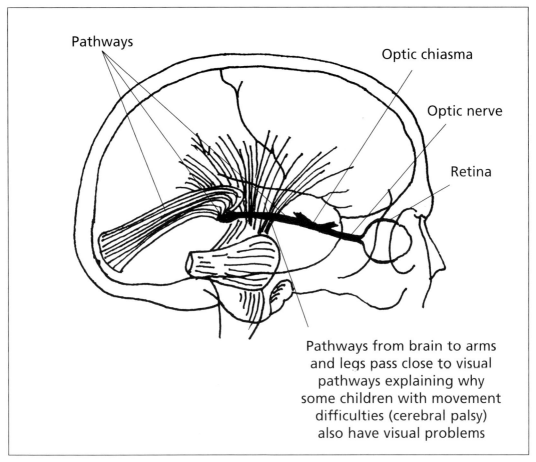

Pathways

Optic chiasma

Optic nerve

Retina

Pathways from brain to arms
and legs pass close to visual
pathways explaining why
some children with movement
difficulties (cerebral palsy)
also have visual problems

translated through increasingly complex interconnections between
brain cells (only a few of which are beginning to be understood) into
our amazingly detailed and colourful perceptions of the visual world.

Visual cortex

The first area of the cortex involved in processing the visual image is
situated at the back of the brain **(see Figures 1.5 and 1.6)** and is
called the primary visual cortex. The first cells in the visual pathway
which respond to input from both eyes are situated here and they
give rise to the ability to join pictures from both eyes (binocular
vision) and perception of depth. The visual system is exquisitely

organised. If you look, for example, at someone's nose, then at the same time your peripheral vision is good enough to register a single left eyebrow hair as a signal in each eye. These two signals are carried to exactly the same cell at the back of the brain in the visual cortex.

Although the majority of visual information does arrive at the cortex of the brain by the route described, there are alternative quicker routes which bypass the cortex and which are important for quick visual reflexes. The way our pupils react instantly to bright light is an obvious example but there may be other pathways which allow reflex responses to visual stimuli. Birds, for instance, flying through trees at high speed require very quick visual responses to avoid crashing. This unconscious awareness (conscious vision only occurs in the cortex) of certain objects, moving or stationary, is present to a more limited degree in humans and is manifested as so-called 'blindsight' (unconscious visual awareness of surroundings) in people with damage to the visual cortex.

Seeing contrast and movement
The brain is arranged in such a way that the electrical signals coming from the eyes are broken down into the components of the picture. The mind detects edges and boundaries, and their shape and orientation. The picture is built up in the mind from its parts.

The imagery is then compared with pictures which have been 'stored' from the past. If the picture which is seen matches with the memory store it is recognised. If it is not recognised then the object is explored with as many senses as possible and a cross-referenced memory map across the different senses is created. This 'cognition' takes place ready for future recognition.

Colour vision
Light is the part of the electromagnetic spectrum which people happen to have receptors for, and it is our minds which are responsible for imparting the concept of colour for each wavelength of light. In the retina we have three types of cell (or cones) each of which absorbs different components of the light coming in. One type

THE BRAIN CONNECTIONS INVOLVED

Edges and borders are what help define shapes and contours in our three dimensional world. The brain is able to 'see' such contrasts by the complex reactions of cells in the retina to light reflected from objects. When light is coming in from a flat surface or uniform colour, all the receptor cells of the retina are stimulated, and send corresponding signals to the visual cortex of the brain, where the signals are translated into the visual images which we 'see'. If the cells are stimulated by an edge ie a border between a lighter shade and a darker one, a stronger signal than that resulting from the uniform stimulus is sent to the visual cortex to be processed. Further levels of complexity of processing mean that some cells respond selectively to vertical and some to horizontal edges, and various others to different orientations between the vertical and horizontal. Other cells (on-off cells) do not respond to a constant light stimulus but only respond if the light is switched on or off. Groups of these cells may be wired to another cell (a movement cell) further along the line of processing, in such a way that a light source moving in a particular direction will sequentially stimulate the on-off cells, and this will be registered as movement by that next cell, the movement cell.

We can therefore see that there is a progression of increasing complexity along the chains of brain cells which begin with the receptors being stimulated by uniform light, but more strongly stimulated by edges and borders. Further along the chain are cells which are stimulated by changes in light, (eg on-off or movement) and it is hypothesised by scientists that as the connections between the cells become increasingly intricate, so some cells will eventually learn to respond to a particular image eg a familiar face. However, although this represents a considerable recent advance in the understanding of the processing of visual information by the brain, the fundamental process by which electrical signals in such cells are ultimately interpreted as the images of the visual world by the 'mind's eye' remains an enigma.

of cone mainly absorbs green, one red and one blue. The colour we see depends on how much each is stimulated by the incoming light. It is no coincidence that the colours of the dots or pixels on a TV screen are matched to the colours seen by our receptors (red, green and blue). Just as any colour can be created on the screen from these pixels, colours can be created in the mind by the signals from the three cone types in our retina. If one of the cone types (usually red or green) is deficient there may be difficulty in distinguishing reds from greens. This is the cause of impaired colour vision in about one in twelve to one in fifteen men.

A separate area at the back of the brain is responsible for processing colours and for *'setting'* the colour balance, so that for all types of lighting, from the pink of the dawn to the black of a thunderstorm, the colour of grass for instance remains green to the mind's eye because the brain *'knows'* that grass is green. This part of the brain can occasionally be damaged, for example by carbon monoxide poisoning. People with such damage see the world clearly but in black and white, like watching black and white TV.

The nature of colour

Imagine a grey ball. Above it is a white ball and below, a black ball, and between them there are balls of all shades of grey arranged in order. The central grey is often used as a base paint in shops supplying paint. If you add red the grey will gradually become redder until it can't become any more red and the hue of red gradually becomes more red until it is fully saturated as a primary colour. (You can't get redder than red.) If you were to do the same with each of the colours you can imagine a circle around the central grey in which red blends into orange, orange into yellow, yellow into green, green into blue and blue through purple back to red again. This is called the colour circle with inner (imaginary) circles of equivalent, washed-out looking desaturated hues. If you now choose to add white or black to say your red hue, you would create either pink (a tint) or brown (a shade) which would ultimately blend into light pink through to white or through dark brown into black. This is what is known as colour contrast. The greater the degree of *'blackness'* or *'whiteness'* present within adjacent colours, the greater the amount of contrast between them and the clearer the boundary between the two colours.

The way that colour vision is coded in the brain means although we can mix certain colours to see for instance a reddish blue (magenta) or a reddish yellow (orange), there are certain colours that cannot be mixed in this way but instead tend to contrast starkly with each other across a colour border. For instance, we can never see a reddish green or a bluish yellow, but yellow writing shows up clearly against a blue background and is a good combination to use in visual aids because of this.

Dark shades absorb light (and get warmer because the energy is converted into heat) and light tints reflect light and feel cooler, in bright sunlight in particular, as less light is absorbed. A blind person can therefore feel a dark colour as truly being warmer to the touch than a light colour when these colours are brightly lit.

Learning to use vision

Increasingly complicated levels of processing and coding of various aspects of an image take place throughout the visual pathways (eg from retina to primary visual cortex and from one area of the visual cortex to another). The primary visual cortex is the first part of the cortex to receive the image and it sends messages to numerous other areas of the cortex (sometimes known as visual association areas) where not only does more complex analysis of the visual information take place but this information can be combined with other sensory information (such as that from touch and hearing), and can be stored in memory so that it becomes the basis for future recognition, imagination and dreams. As visual information is continually arriving, it is compared and matched with the information already stored in the memory bank. A pattern match leads to recognition and reinforcement. If the incoming information has not been met before and has not been stored in the memory bank, no match can occur. The information will then be learned, so that if met again, it will be recognised. Repeated viewing enhances recall but lack of such reinforcement makes subsequent recognition more difficult. Damage to the brain responsible for this highly complex system of information storage, retrieval and matching can therefore cause impairment of vision at an intellectual level. Children with multiple disabilities due to brain damage may show evidence of a wide range of such intellectual or 'cognitive' visual disorders, many of which remain to be classified

COLOUR CONFUSION
(often inaccurately labelled colour blindness - Plate 3)

Some people are completely lacking in one of the three types of cone systems. Although their world does not appear black and white they do experience a smaller variety of colours. These people are called dichromats (meaning 'two colours'). A more common type of colour confusion is called anomalous colour vision which means that although such people require mixtures of three coloured lights to make their colours, they use different proportions and therefore see colours differently from those with normal colour vision. Two colours matched as identical by someone with normal colour vision may also be seen as identical by a dichromat but may look different to someone with anomalous colour vision.

Red-green colour confusion is surprisingly common with around eight per cent of men markedly deficient, though it is extremely rare in women because it is inherited in an X-linked fashion (see Glossary). Anomalous (incomplete) red-green confusion is more common (6%) than dichromatic (complete) red-green confusion (2%). The Ishihara colour plates (to be discussed more fully in Chapter 2) were designed to test for and distinguish the specific types of inherited colour confusions mentioned above. These inherited forms of colour confusion do not constitute visual impairment and studies have shown that children are not adversely affected by it in educational terms.

Colour vision defects can also be caused by a variety of diseases that damage the retina, optic nerve or visual cortex. Although such deficiencies do not fall into the neat colour categories above (because, for example all three types of cone might be affected) there is a tendency for macular disorders to cause more blue-yellow confusion and for optic nerve disorders to cause more red-green confusion. With increasing severity of the disease the defect tends to affect all types of colour discrimination.

and understood, but this should not prevent us from having a very open mind when caring for children with problems of this nature.

FIGURE 1.6 - *Specialised areas of the brain*

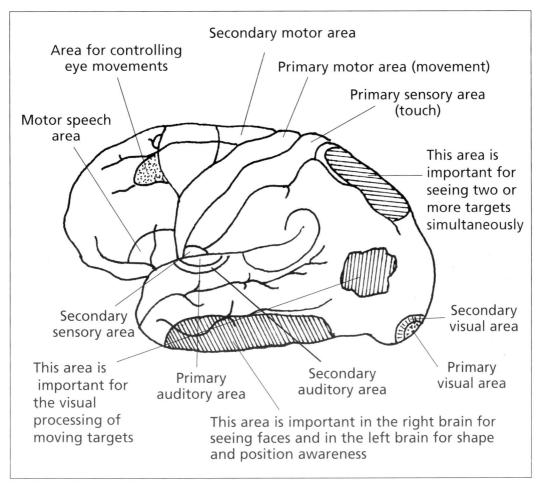

Figure 1.6 shows some examples of specialised areas of visual cortex (sometimes called visual association cortex) including those with particular responsibility for the processing of motion and face and shape recognition. These areas are only beginning to be recognised and understood. Some of these types of processing occur on both sides of the brain (eg colour and motion perception) whereas other types tend to occur predominantly on one side. For example, damage to the left side of the brain may lead to poor appreciation of internal detail of an object, whereas damage to the right side may lead to poor appreciation of the outline and orientation of an object. The left

side of the brain seems to be important for reading and recognising shapes, and the right side of the brain seems to be important for recognising faces, and for the ability to work out where we are and to find our way and to know where we have put things.

Another example of higher visual function processing involves speech. In most right-handed people speech is processed in the left side of the brain. There is one (sensory) centre where the brain receives and processes speech and language information and another (motor) centre where our own speech originates **(see Figure 1.7)**. The sensory speech area is situated close to the visual association cortex (as well as to the corresponding auditory association cortex). Different parts of visual association cortex process the visual information about mouth movements and facial expressions of a person who is speaking, or about written words as they are read, and they send this information to the nearby sensory speech and language area.

A similar process operates for the corresponding auditory association areas, where the sounds of spoken words are processed. The sensory speech area having received all this information, then integrates and interprets it and sends signals on through a bundle of nerve fibres to the motor centre where corresponding speech is initiated. Visually impaired children lack the visual experience of facial expressions and mouth movements which accompany various spoken words and therefore their whole concept of the meaning of words and the way in which they learn such meaning is affected, making it important to use *'larger than life'* expressions, gestures and signs and body language. Such stimulation needs of course to be within the measured capacity of the child to see, which highlights the importance of regular assessment of the functional vision and working well within the child's limits.

In the future, increasing knowledge of the specialised functions of different areas of the brain will no doubt aid our understanding of the particular learning difficulties encountered by children with brain damage in these areas.

FIGURE 1.7 - *Diagram showing the probable nervous pathways involved in reading a sentence and repeating it aloud.*

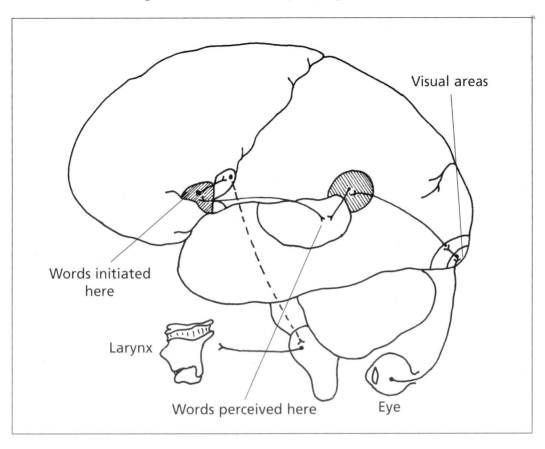

We have said that for visual perception to become meaningful, images must be compared with those previously experienced. In order for visual (or indeed any sensory) memory to be laid down there must be an element of *'plasticity'* of the connections between brain cells throughout life. What this means is that not all the wiring patterns between brain cells are established at birth, but rather that these connections are established and then reinforced by repeated stimulation during early life. Thus the process of learning through repetition can be thought of as giving rise to the laying down of wiring patterns between sets of brain cells. This process is maximal during childhood but continues into old age. A simple example of the importance of this in early life is found by returning to visual cortical cells. Certain of these cells each respond to a line of a particular orientation.

It has been shown that if a kitten is reared in an environment of vertical lines only, then no brain cells will develop which will respond to edges in other orientations. If the kitten is reared in complete darkness then this response to edges may fail to develop completely. Such sensitivity of the brain to visual disturbance is known to be greatest in young children, and if the young child's visual system is deprived of well focused images, then permanent visual impairment may develop at the level of the visual cortex, even if the focusing problem is later resolved (hence the importance of diagnosing and treating all causes of treatable visual impairment at an early age). This condition in which the brain does not develop the capacity to see well owing to the poor quality of the pictures presented to it during early life is called deprivational amblyopia.

The implication of this plasticity of the young visual system is that every effort should be made to stimulate vision fully from an early age. This will mean different strategies for different children. Those children with cataracts, for instance, may need surgery at a very young age and then encouragement to wear their glasses or contact lenses as much of the time as possible; children with one damaged eye and one healthy eye may need the healthy eye to be patched for a number of hours every day to encourage development of the pathways from the damaged eye; and visually impaired children for whom no surgical or optical intervention may be possible should be provided with visually interesting stimuli to maximise the signals which are sent from the eyes to the brain in order to optimise the development of these pathways.

CHAPTER 2

ASSESSMENT AND MEASUREMENT OF VISION

This chapter is concerned with how various aspects of vision can be measured and assessed. It aims to clarify how the measurements are made and what they mean in the context of the child's understanding and education. When a doctor, optician or orthoptist tests vision, it is usually to find out how well each eye is functioning. This is either to make a diagnosis or to follow up the vision after treatment. For this reason the test is usually carried out at a distance (which detects people who are short sighted) and for each eye in turn.

It is essential that teachers and parents working with a child who is visually impaired are able to understand what the child can and cannot see. There is no point in using educational material which has images which are too small to be seen and are therefore *'not there'*. (Look at woven cloth through a magnifying glass. The fine detail of the weave which was *'not there'* before suddenly becomes apparent and has significance.) For this reason we are not interested in what each eye sees independently and the clarity of vision in the distance is only one of many factors. It is therefore important to be able to *'test'* vision with both eyes open, and to assess near and distance vision for acuity, colour contrast, visual fields, optimum lighting conditions and movement perception. Educational material is of limited or no value if parts or all of it cannot be seen by the child. The child *'knows'* that his or her vision is *'normal'*. Just as you accept as *'normal'* your inability to see detail, the further away you are, children with reduced vision are unaware of what they are missing and accept this as *'normal'*. This is why it is so important for teachers to be aware of what various assessments of vision mean in terms of what is accessible to a child and what is not, and to be aware of which components of educational material can and cannot be seen by children.

HISTORY TAKING

Before looking at the various techniques for measuring vision it must be remembered that a lot of information can be gained about various aspects of the child's functional vision from talking to the child and parents. Indeed the parents may well have picked up much more useful information about educationally relevant aspects of the child's visual impairment from years of living with him or her, than a doctor can elicit from a relatively short consultation in the somewhat artificial environment of the clinic.

It is our opinion that before a child comes into a school or class for the first time, the teacher should spend a considerable time talking to the parents, asking questions and learning from their vast experience of the child's visual functions and problems. The art of 'history taking' (the name doctors give to the process of eliciting useful information from talking to patients and families) is learned by the practice of doing it throughout a career. An important element is the use of the specialist information that the interviewer, in this case the teacher, has gained from training and from experience with other children with similar problems. This should enable the interviewer to ask specific questions with the aim of identifying or eliminating specific visual problems or strengths which the child might be exhibiting. The parents may well have an impression of these problems or strengths but may have difficulty articulating them accurately without prompting from specific expert questioning. Another reason that this detailed interview is important is that although we may be very familiar with the sort of problems to expect in a child with albinism for instance, both from our reading and our experience, we know that no two children with albinism will have exactly the same visual problems to the same degree. Thus the interview with the parents is a good source of information about the individual capacities and requirements of that particular child.

This sort of interview should be repeated regularly because the visual abilities and disabilities of any child may not be static. Repeating the interviews may therefore elicit new and useful information from the parents while also conveying the message to them that change and progress are generally to be sought and expected.

We propose a possible structure for questions covering the principal aspects of functional vision but a teacher may want to develop her own set of questions to be modified in the light of experience.

1. Introductory questions

Opening questions should be very general so as not to bias the parents' responses. For example 'What do you think your child can and cannot see?' or 'How well do you think he or she can see?' or 'Do you have any particular concerns about your child's vision?' The answers to these general questions may affect the further direction of the interview with more detailed and directed questions being addressed to particular problems or strengths identified by the parents.

2. Peripheral vision

As explained in Chapter 1, this is particularly important for navigation and therefore the sort of questions to ask would be 'How does he manage to get around the room or house?' 'Does she bump into things much?' Children with cortical visual impairment often see better on one side (hemianopia). 'Does she see better on the right or left?' 'Does she bump into things more on the right or left?' 'Does he have to move his head to the left or right to look there?' Answers to such questions may have obvious implications for positioning in the classroom. It should be realised that unusual head movements or postures may not be indicative of a peripheral visual deficit but can occur in eye movement disorders. For instance, wobble of the eyes (nystagmus) can be reduced, hence improving vision, by the adoption of a particular head posture in some children. Other children may be able to eliminate double vision by holding their head in a certain way. Adoption of such head postures should not be discouraged.

3. Central, detailed vision (visual acuity)

This can be ascertained, perhaps, by asking the parents to bring in books or pictures which they know that the child responds to. The smaller and more detailed a text or picture which the child favours, the better is the functional acuity. It will usually be found that the material favoured by a child will be larger than might be suggested by the 'official' acuity, which by definition is the smallest detail which the child can possibly see (not what he or she can comfortably and easily see in practice).

4. Near and distance vision

'How far does he sit from the TV?' 'How close does she hold books or toys to her eyes?' 'Does she seem to see better for near or for distance?' Certain conditions are associated with better near than distance vision (eg myopia, albinism) and others with better distant vision than near (eg macular disorders). Answers to such questions again may help positioning in the classroom or may give clues about which if any Low Vision Aids (LVAs) might be helpful for a particular child (eg text may be held very close, not because a child is short sighted, but to magnify it, see **Figure 2.2**).

5. Lighting conditions

'How does he see in the dark?' 'Does bright sunlight bother her?' 'Does he prefer general lighting or lighting for a specific task?' Different children with different conditions will give different answers to these questions.

6. Three dimensional vision

'How does she cope with steps and kerbs?' This is a problem which we have encountered in a number of children with cortical visual impairment who see steps and kerbs just as lines on the ground. This is relevant not only to classroom set-up (eg marking steps clearly) but also to the type of educational material used (since 3D objects may be seen as flat).

7.   Colour vision

'Are some colours seen better than others?' 'Does she have favourite colours?' As explained later in this chapter, the objective tests used for assessing colour vision are often not designed with visually impaired children in mind and direct questioning can therefore be quite useful. Again, educational materials can then be tailored to the individual child. Children learn to match colours before they can name them. If naming is a problem, questions about how well colours are matched are appropriate.

8.   Specific disorders

A whole range of specific visual challenges occur in a variety of conditions, some of which are outlined in Chapter 3 and which the teacher might specifically enquire about if the diagnosis is known. The best examples probably occur in cortical visual impairment where a number of different functional deficits are now beginning to be recognised. These can sometimes be quite subtle and not elicited unless you specifically ask about them. Examples include difficulties knowing how to 'see' where one is and how to move to a new location, difficulty recognising faces and failure to see fast-moving objects. More is said about these problems in Chapter 3.

REFRACTION

The measurement of the correct lenses required to bring the images seen by the eyes into best focus is known as refraction. All children with reduced vision should be refracted, and testing of vision carried out with the child wearing the correct spectacles, unless of course this is impracticable.

Refraction is the specialist field of optometrists, though it is also commonly performed for children by ophthalmologists. It can be carried out subjectively in children who are old and able enough to co-operate. This is the procedure familiar to any of us who have our eyes tested at high street optometrists where the person being tested informs the tester whether particular lenses improve or worsen the clarity of vision until the best strength of lens is found. If the child is too young or is unable to co-operate, the refraction can be performed objectively, a process involving the observation of a moving reflected light on the retina. This technique is known as retinoscopy.

FIGURE 2.1- *Normal sight, short sight (myopia), long sight (hypermetropia)*

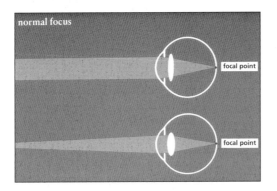
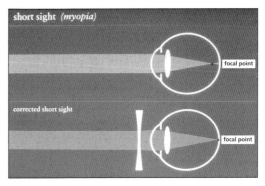
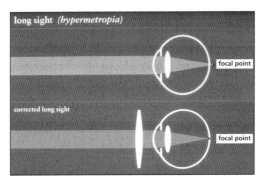

RETINOSCOPY

In young children, eye drops which paralyse the ability of the eye to focus are used. A technique known as retinoscopy (objective refraction) is then used to find out which lenses are needed. **Figure 2.1** shows that a short sighted eye brings light to a focus in front of the retina and that a lower ray hits the upper retina, but in a long sighted eye this ray hits the lower retina. The view through a retinoscope is the same as for a flash photograph. A red glow is seen in the pupil. When the retinoscope moves, the red glow moves. In short sighted eyes the red glow moves in the opposite direction to the movement of the retinoscope (because the light rays cross inside the eye) but in long sighted eyes the red glow moves in the same direction as the retinoscope is moving. So all the refractionist (optician or ophthalmologist) has to do is to find out which lens in front of the eye is accompanied by no movement of the red glow. From this knowledge the lens required is calculated. Older children and adults are asked which lens suits them best in a structured process of trial and error known as subjective refraction.

Early diagnosis and correction of refractive errors is very important in young children because a blurred image on the developing retina causes amblyopia as already described in Chapter 1.

REFRACTIVE ERRORS

Figure 2.1 is a simple ray diagram of the way the eye focuses light onto the retina. The curvature and consistency of the cornea and the lens determine their *'power'* as optical lenses which means the degree to which they bend light rays. **Figure 2.1** shows that for light to be focused into a sharp point image on the retina, the power of the cornea and lens need to be matched exactly with the length of the eyeball. It is a mismatch between these two factors, (the optical power and the length of the eye) which gives rise to the two commonest refractive errors, short sightedness (myopia) and long sightedness (hypermetropia). **Figure 2.1** also shows that if the focusing power of the eye is too powerful (ie the eyeball is too long and short sighted) then the image is formed in front of the retina and the image at the retina will be blurred because it is out of focus. Increased focusing power is needed to see near targets (see accommodation) so that a short sighted eye is in focus for near, hence the term. The nearer an object has to be brought towards the eyes for it to be seen clearly, the more short sighted the person is. The closer something is to the eye, the bigger it appears **(Figure 2.2)**. This means that a short sighted child with an additional cause of poor vision may choose to remove his glasses and view what he is looking at from close up, which makes it look bigger. This has the same effect as using a magnifying glass, giving higher magnification with a narrower field of view.

FIGURE 2.2 - *The closer an object is to the eye, the larger it appears*

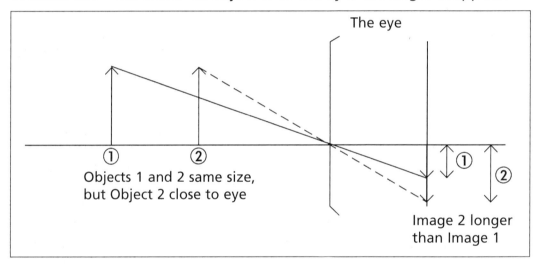

In long sightedness the opposite occurs **(see Figure 2.1)**. The focusing power is too weak and the eyeball is relatively short, so objects further away may be seen more clearly than near ones. Often, glasses are not prescribed for small amounts of long sightedness because the focusing power of the eye compensates for the long sight by bringing the image into focus.

Refractive error and squint: We can focus using accommodation to overcome long sightedness and children, in particular, have good focusing power. So mild to moderate degrees of long sightedness do not blur vision in children. However, whenever we look at something which is close to us we also turn our eyes in (they converge). The two reflexes of focusing (or accommodation) and turning in (or converging) are closely linked. A long sighted child has to accommodate without turning the eyes in. If he can't do this then the long sightedness causes the eye to turn in, resulting in a convergent squint. Convergent squint due to long sight is common. Children with brain damage may have difficulty in focusing to overcome long sightedness without at the same time turning their eyes in. Relatively minor degrees of long sightedness may be the cause of convergent squint in such children. The provision of glasses may therefore be required to straighten the eyes rather than to make vision clearer.

When an eye turns in, the brain may choose to neglect the image from that eye, with resultant poorer vision or amblyopia. Patching the 'good' eye may be required to reverse this process and to restore vision in the squinting eye.

Astigmatism: Another common refractive error is called astigmatism. For accurate focusing of light the optical surfaces should be smoothly and regularly curved like the surface of a perfect sphere. Astigmatism simply means that the optical surface (usually the cornea) is not spherical but has different curvatures in different orientations (rather like the curvature of a rugby ball compared to a football). It is easy to imagine how the image of a three dimensional object is distorted by this situation. The lens required to correct astigmatism has a reciprocal rugby ball shaped curve aligned at 90 degrees to the rugby ball curve alignment of the surface of the cornea.

Refractive errors can usually be compensated for by placing optical lenses in front of the eyes in the form of spectacles or contact lenses **(see Figure 2.1)**.

VISUAL ACUITY

Simply, this means the ability to see fine detail and is one of the most important and commonly recorded measurements of visual function. This ability to see detail depends on a number of different factors which must be taken into account when measuring acuity. Such factors include the level of background illumination, the contrast of the target against its background (eg it is easier to see a black letter on a white background than a dark grey letter on a lighter grey background), the distance between eye and the target, and whether a refractive error is present (and if so whether it has been accurately corrected with lenses).

FIGURE 2.3a - *Distance visual acuity: Snellen charts - the visual acuity measure is normally based on the line of letters/symbols which can be read at 6m. The small numbers (enlarged on left) refer to the distance at which a normal eye can read the letter. Subjects who cannot read the top letter at 6m will be tested closer to the chart.*

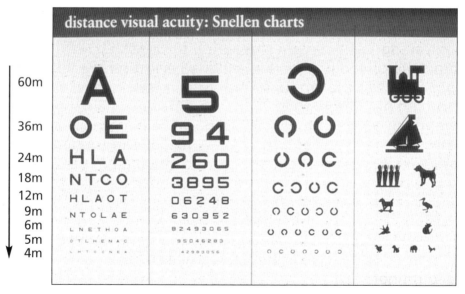

The commonest way of measuring visual acuity is to use the Snellen Chart **(Figure 2.3a)** at six metres distance away **(Figure 2.3b)**. This is based on the principle that an object of fixed size gives a smaller image on the retina the further away it is viewed. Conversely objects of different sizes can give the same size of image on the retina if viewed from different distances **(Figure 2.2)**. The chart, shown on the left in **Figure 2.3a**, consists of rows of black letters on a white background. The upper row of letters is the largest and is said to be seen by a normal eye at a distance of sixty metres away. The smallest sized letters are on the lowest line and are said to be readable by a normal eye at five metres away. The letters of the top row when viewed from sixty metres give an image on the retina which is the same size as the image of the letters on the bottom line when they are viewed from five metres.

The visual acuity is recorded as a fraction, the numerator or first number of the fraction being the distance that the chart is placed from the eye in metres (most commonly six) and the denominator or second part of the fraction denoting the smallest (lowest) line which can be read by the eye at six metres (in other words the distance from which a normal eye could see that line). The large top letter on the chart can just be made out at a distance of sixty metres. So, for instance, an eye which could only read the top letter of the chart at six metres would be said to have an acuity of six over sixty (or six sixty), meaning that what a normal eye could read from sixty metres away this eye can only see from six metres away. This can be thought of as six sixtieths or ten percent of normal visual acuity.

In theory the smallest line a normal eye would be able to read at six metres would be the six metre line and would be recorded as having an acuity of six six (In the USA the chart is situated twenty feet away and hence the term 'twenty twenty' for perfect acuity.) In practice however, the standards of the chart err on the generous side and most normal eyes can read the smaller five metre line at six metres. Hence a perfect visual acuity is closer to six five than to six six.

If a child cannot read even the top letter at six metres, ie the acuity is worse than six sixty, then the child can be moved closer to the chart until the top letter can be seen. If the top letter can be seen at three metres, the acuity would be recorded as three over sixty; if it is not seen until the child is one metre away then the acuity would be one over sixty. If the top letter cannot be seen at all then poor visual acuities are conventionally classified into the ability to count fingers (this can be subdivided into the distance at which the child can count fingers again from one to six metres, often abbreviated to eg CF at 1m); the ability to detect movement of a hand (HM); the ability to perceive light (PL); and no ability to perceive light (NPL).

FIGURE 2.3b - *Distance visual acuity: Snellen charts - the child is reading the Snellen chart (back to front as above) with his left eye via a mirror facing him 3 metres away so that the total distance is 6 metres.*

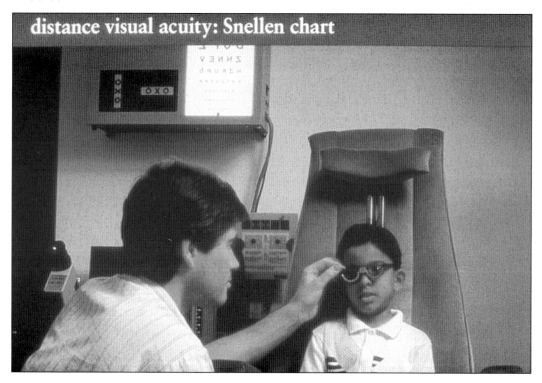

The two eyes are normally tested separately by ophthalmologists and opticians, but functional vision is best tested with both eyes open and may be one line better than either of the two monocular acuities.

Obviously, to use the Snellen chart requires that a child can read, recognise and verbalise the letters on the chart. Variations of the Snellen chart have therefore been devised for younger, preverbal children or for those with learning difficulties. The Landolt ring **(Figure 2.3a)**, Illiterate E chart and Lea heart-shape chart require the child to detect the orientation of a particular figure and to match it with a similarly orientated figure from a selection of figures of various orientations contained on a smaller chart held in their hand. Pictures instead of figures **(Figure 2.3a)**, can also be identified or matched as in the Kay's picture test.

Even these adaptations require a measure of co-operation from the child and for very young children or those with severe learning difficulties an attempt to estimate their acuity can be made either with electrical measurements, as explained in a later section of this chapter, or with a technique called the acuity card procedure which relies on the principle of preferential looking. This latter technique relies on the finding that if a child is presented with two visual targets, one plain and one patterned, then the child will reflexly look towards the patterned target. This is thought to arise from the visual system's built-in preference for contrast and edges (see Contrast and movement, Chapter 1). Thus the test involves the child being presented with a series of large cards each containing two target areas, one plain grey and one with black and white stripes. The assessor observes the child's eye movements through a small hole in the card and decides which way the child is looking. The size of the stripes is gradually reduced and below a certain size corresponding to the child's limit of resolution or acuity, the black and white stripes will just appear as a grey blur and the fixation preference will be lost. A variation of this test for slightly older children involves Cardiff cards **(Plate 4)**. These are rectangular cards which are presented vertically with a picture at the top or bottom. The picture is bounded by a zebra like line which is made up of black and white stripes. The card is presented in front of the child and his eyes are observed to see if they move to look at the picture. Successive cards are shown in which the boundary line gets finer and finer until it can no longer be seen and the black and white images merge into the central grey and the picture effectively disappears. This is one of the best tests of acuity for young school age children and pre-school children.

A common misconception is to confuse the concepts of refractive error and acuity and hence to equate six six or twenty twenty vision with someone who does not need glasses. In fact, visual acuity should always be recorded with glasses on if they are needed; most of the spectacle wearing population do have acuities of six six or six five with their glasses on and are obviously not considered to be visually impaired.

Another misconception to be aware of is equating visual acuity with vision. The ability to see fine detail is a very important aspect of vision but is not the only one - it involves the central macular area of the retina and the central part of the visual field (see next section). It is therefore quite possible for a child with retinitis pigmentosa for example, to have acuities of six six in each eye but to have severe tunnel vision and difficulty seeing in poor light and so to be significantly visually impaired. Conversely, a child with a disease of both maculae (for example cone dystrophy) may have a poor acuity but minimal impairment of mobility owing to intact peripheral vision. **Plates 5-7** attempt to simulate the perception of blurred focus due to an uncorrected refractive error and reduced visual acuity.

FUNCTIONAL ACUITY

It is important to realize that the official Snellen acuity fraction that is recorded in the clinic may not correlate simply with the functional acuity in the home or the classroom. The level of illumination in a room in fact has surprisingly little effect on acuity (as long as there is enough light for cone stimulation) - visual acuity remains constant over a wide range of lighting levels extending from the level of full moonlight to that of a bright sky on a sunny day. However, although clarity may not be reduced by lower light levels, the time taken to perceive fine detail is prolonged as background lighting is reduced. This is very important for schools where the time taken to accomplish a task is important. (See section on Lighting in Chapter 4.)

Other factors such as the spacing of visual targets or the distance from which they are viewed may have more significant effects on whether they can be clearly seen. These factors can be regulated in the clinic but not always in the real-life situation of home or classroom.

Visual acuity can be reduced in children when targets are presented too close together. This phenomenon is known as *crowding* and is particularly noticeable in children with amblyopia or cortical visual impairment. Indeed, the Snellen chart suffers from a degree of inaccuracy because the spacing between the letters varies on different lines. An eye with amblyopia in particular will score significantly better on modified Snellen charts with only one letter on each line.

Contrast is another factor to be considered. This will be described in greater detail in the section on contrast sensitivity but it is worth emphasising that visual acuity is a measure of the ability to discriminate detail in targets of maximum contrast such as black letters on a white background. The visual targets in the child's everyday environment may not be seen in such ideal black and white contrast conditions. Finally, it must be remembered that Snellen acuities are measured at six metres and therefore represent an assessment of distance vision. It is often, however, objects at close range which require detailed visual discrimination. There is a strong correlation between near and distance visual acuity but there are conditions where one is significantly better than the other. Disorders of the macula, for instance, although adversely affecting both near and distant acuities sometimes have more of an adverse effect on the near acuity. Conversely, nystagmus (wobbling eyes) is reduced and the eyes wobble less when they turn in or converge to look at a near target, giving better near vision. **Plate 8** attempts to simulate the effect of nystagmus on visual perception.

Because of these differences it is often helpful to measure formally the near visual acuity with a near reading chart containing print of different sizes and record both at the normal comfortable reading distance, and in the position that the child normally chooses to adopt. The tests available are poorly standardized and include reduced

Snellen charts, Maclure charts **(Figure 2.4)** and the Point and Jaeger charts. These may use letters, unrelated words or meaningful text. Near acuity is a better predictor of the optimum magnification for visually impaired readers than distance acuity and is a better predictor of educational performance than distance acuity. A better predictive test still is to observe the ease and speed of periods of sustained reading of different sized prints in the school environment.

The near acuity as measured in the eye clinic involves only reading a few words and the very smallest that can be read (often with difficulty) will be recorded. Obviously this should on no account be taken as the optimum print size for educational material, which should be well within rather than at the child's visual limits.

FIGURE 2.4 - *Near visual acuity: Maclure chart test*

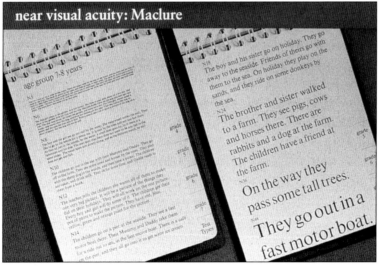

Older children with milder forms of visual impairment may be considering learning to drive. There are strict criteria issued by the medical advisers to the DVLC on minimum acuities and visual fields for safe driving. The visual acuity criteria require the ability to read a car number plate at a distance of 20.5 metres (with glasses if needed) and this is included in the driving test itself. This cannot simply be translated into a Snellen acuity recorded in the clinic for the reasons outlined above (conditions outside are not idealized as in the clinic: for example, glare may be a problem and the number plate may not be black against white), but the nearest estimate is in the region of six over twelve in the better eye. The visual field criteria which must be met are not included in the driving test and are described in the next section. Another aspect of functional vision of relevance to education is the concept of dynamic acuity, which is simply a measure of the visual acuity when either the target or the person is moving. This has been the subject of small studies mainly in sportsmen and women; eye muscle coordination is thought to be important in the ability to localise accurately and quickly, and to resolve the detail of moving targets. Children with eye movement disorders, which cause difficulty in tracking moving objects, can have reduced clarity of vision for moving targets, and may, for example, have impaired ability in extracting visual information from films and videos - particularly fast moving cartoons. Such children are typically those with cerebral palsy who may also have cortical visual impairment.

Rarely, children with cortical visual impairment may have damage on both sides of the part of the brain responsible for seeing movement. These children appear not to see moving targets unless they are moving very slowly, yet their clarity of vision may even be normal. It is as if the whole moving world blurs out. This condition is called akinetopsia.

VISUAL FIELDS

This concept was introduced in Chapter 1. The visual field is the proportion of space around us which is visible at any one moment. **Figure 2.5a** and **Plate 9** show the normal boundaries of the visual fields. Assessing visual fields involves measuring these boundaries (ie finding out how far right, left, up or down an eye can see while looking straight ahead) and also measuring how sensitive the vision is (eg how small a target or dim a light can be seen) at various places within these boundaries. Formal mapping of the visual field involves the child looking at a central target on a screen **(Plate 9)**. Points of light of various size and brightness are then momentarily flashed up on the screen at different positions on the screen, and the subject indicates if they have been seen. In this way a map of the visual field is built up as shown in **Plate 9.**

FIGURE 2.5a - *The visual field of each eye is cut off by the nose. The extreme right field of vision is seen by the right eye only and the extreme left field of vision by the left eye only. (Diagram shows view from above.)*

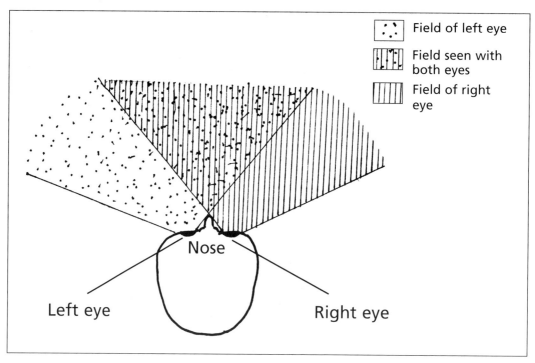

There are various computerised machines available for performing visual field tests and analysing the results, but these sophisticated tests usually take a long time to perform and are also quite difficult even for adult patients. They are therefore of limited use in children, though some child-friendly versions are being developed using the type of graphics used in computer games.

Simpler methods can give an estimate of visual field boundaries; eg one adult engages the child's visual attention while another introduces a toy into the edge of the child's vision noting when the child turns his head to look at it. This can easily be done at home or in the classroom and provides a very useful idea of the true functional field of vision **(Plate 10)**. However, a negative test must be treated with caution and repeated because the central target can be so

interesting to the child that everything else is ignored.
Sensitivity decreases in all directions away from the point of fixation
and hence the visual field can be imagined as a meringue shaped
island or hill of vision in a sea of blindness. As mentioned in Chapter 1
and shown in **Figure 2.5b** the normal visual field of each eye contains
a blind spot corresponding to the optic nerve head where there are
no photoreceptors (see **Figure 2.6** to demonstrate your own blind
spot). With both eyes open there is no blind spot since the field of one
eye covers the blind spot of the other eye. This normal blind spot is

FIGURE 2.5b - *3D map of visual field of right eye*

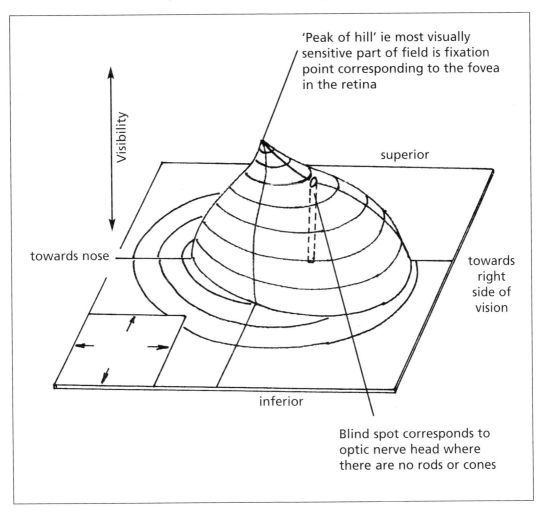

an example of what is termed a scotoma, an area of reduced light sensitivity. Scotomata other than the normal blind spot are due to disorders of the eye or visual pathway, and indeed the pattern of the scotoma may indicate where in the eye or visual pathway the disorder is located. Scotomata may be absolute (no light perception in that area) or relative (reduced, but not absent, light sensitivity). Scotomata can also be classified as 'positive' when they are noticed as a shadow obscuring part of the visual field (eg a retinal detachment is often initially seen as a grey curtain-like shadow over part of the vision), or 'negative' when they are not noticed as a shadow (such as the blind spot or the various scotomata which result from damage to areas of the visual brain) but in which vision is reduced or absent.

FIGURE 2.6 - *The normal blind spot. Close your left eye and look at the cross with the right. Hold the page close to your eye and slowly move it away keeping your eye fixed on the cross. The dot will disappear when it reaches the point in space corresponding to your right eye's blind spot. If you open the left eye it will appear again - with both eyes open we do not have a blind spot.*

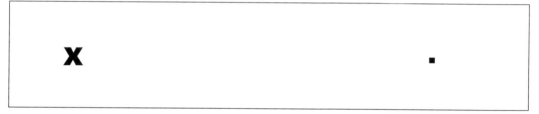

Some of the most common characteristic field losses associated with various visual impairments are represented in **Plates 11-16**. The best known example is probably the progressive closing in of the visual fields seen in retinitis pigmentosa. In severe cases this can lead to very narrow tunnel-like visual fields or even complete extinction of the fields and ultimately, blindness. The child with such severe field restriction may still have a reasonable visual acuity and may therefore be able to read, but perception of the visual world is severely limited to this narrow tunnel of vision with profoundly impaired appreciation of or navigation through the surroundings of the home or classroom, and inability to detect visual events that occur anywhere outside the tiny intact central visual field. Damage to the central retina (for example a macular dystrophy) gives almost a mirror image of this type of tunnel vision field defect, with a centrally located scotoma affecting the central fixation point (as explained in Chapter 1, on the retinal map of visual space, the macula represents the fixation target). Because of its central location such a scotoma is likely to have a profound effect on acuity and the ability to read, while the child's general awareness of her environment and ability to navigate through it will be relatively unimpaired.

Another common form of visual field loss involves one complete half (left or right) of the visual field of both eyes. This is called a homonymous (meaning it is the same side of the field that is affected in each eye) hemianopia (meaning half blind) and is illustrated in **Plate 15**. Behind the optic chiasm or crossover, all the visual information from the left side of the visual field of both eyes travels together in the visual pathways in the right side of the brain, and likewise all the visual information from the right side of the visual field of both eyes travels together in the visual pathways in the left side of the brain. Hence any abnormality (whatever the cause) which affects the right visual brain will tend to cause a left homonymous hemianopia, and any abnormality affecting the left visual brain will tend to cause a right homonymous hemianopia.

It is very important for parents, teachers and mobility specialists to be aware of this type of field defect; only one side of the child's visual world is functioning and obviously all visual interaction should be directed to take place from that side. If you imagine reading print such as this with a hemianopia, the print would suddenly appear out of nowhere for a right hemianopia and suddenly disappear into nowhere for a left hemianopia as the eyes scan across the text. Children with hemianopias may therefore find it easier and eventually faster to tilt the page and read in a direction nearer to the vertical so that the print does not keep appearing or disappearing like this. This technique of reading however requires practice, and acceptance by parents and teachers as being a reasonable and appropriate reading strategy. This provides an example of where the need to conform with what is 'normal' comes into conflict with what may ultimately prove a much faster and more efficient way of accessing information. Chinese is much easier to read!

Because homonymous hemianopia commonly impairs one side of the vision completely it can be tested by a method termed confrontation. The child and examiner face each other and the child is asked to look at the examiner's nose. The examiner then holds up two or three fingers of each hand momentarily so that the examiner can see them in his left and right peripheral vision simultaneously - the child is simply asked how many fingers were held up each side and a significant visual weakness on one side will soon be revealed. The test may be converted into a game where the child is encouraged to look at or grasp the finger which moves. In younger or less cooperative children, lack of head or eye movement to the side of the moving peripheral target suggests that a hemianopia may be present. Children with impaired movement on one side (hemiplegia) often have homonymous hemianopia on the same side.

Children with optic nerve disease may have interrupted visual fields; as though they are looking through a colander as shown in **Plate 16**.

Returning to the question of driving, it is obviously important for drivers to have reasonably good peripheral vision so that they can see a child running out from the pavement, or a cyclist. Therefore people with significant hemianopia or tunnel vision are not allowed to drive even if they have perfect visual acuities. There are strict guidelines issued by the British Licensing Authorities on the minimum degrees of peripheral vision allowable for driving. Any visually impairing condition must be declared to the licensing authority and if there is a question over adequate peripheral vision this can be formally tested in an ophthalmology clinic. The test is performed with both eyes open and therefore someone who is completely blind in one eye but has a full field of vision in the other eye should meet the standard required for a private licence. There are obviously stricter criteria in terms of both acuity and field for issuing licences for professional drivers of heavy goods vehicles or public transport vehicles.

CONTRAST SENSITIVITY

Contrast sensitivity is the ability to discriminate shades of grey, one from the other, while colour contrast sensitivity is the ability to distinguish varying shades of colour - for example light blue from a darker blue. Good contrast sensitivity is required, for example, to be able to make out people's facial features.

Contrast sensitivity can be tested in a number of different ways. In the laboratory, stripes of light and dark grey are made progressively lighter and darker (ie more contrasting) until they can be seen. However there are useful, more practical tests available **(Plate 17)**.

Any condition which impairs central vision, whether it be in the eye, the optic nerve or the brain can impair the ability to detect low contrast. The ability to discriminate contrast is as important as the ability to tell one colour from the other.

ELECTRICAL TESTS OF VISION

Tests of visual function require a degree of cooperation by the child and the results are therefore affected by the child's ability and inclination to perform set tasks. With very young children or those with severe learning difficulties, such tests may be impossible. A more objective test of visual capability involves measurement of the electrical signals being sent along the visual pathways. Electrodes which pick up these electrical signals can be placed on the lower eyelids or on the head over the visual brain areas. The two types of such electrical test which are most often of clinical use are the electroretinogram (ERG) and the visual evoked potential (VEP). The ERG, as its name suggests, measures the electrical signals generated by the retina. These signals are picked up at the front of the eye from an electrode made of silver or gold which is attached to a contact lens or is tucked inside the lid, or is attached to the lower eyelid **(Plate 18)**. The retinal signals are measured in response to a number of different light stimuli to give different information. When the test is performed in bright lighting, the cones of the retina are generating the electrical signal. After the subject has been in the dark for twenty minutes, it is the rods (responsible for night vision) which are being tested. An ERG picked up from someone who is watching a moving black and white chequer board is testing the cells (ganglion cells) which conduct the electrical signals to the brain.

The conditions in which the ERG is most commonly useful are the rod and cone disorders. For instance retinitis pigmentosa predominantly affects the rods and hence the dark-adapted ERG is more affected than the light-adapted ERG.

The VEP involves sticking skin electrodes on to the scalp at the back of the head over the seeing brain or primary visual cortex. Flashes of light or patterned stimuli are again used and the size of the electrical signal generated by the primary visual cortex in response to the pattern is measured and, importantly, any prolongation of the normal one tenth of a second delay between the stimulus and the signal formation in the brain is sought. (We all live one tenth of a second in the past!)

Any disorder at any point along the visual pathway from cornea to visual cortex itself can cause a reduction or a delay in the cortical signal and hence the VEP is a much less specific diagnostic tool than the ERG. VEPs can be useful in telling the difference between a child with a physical disorder in the visual pathway and a child who appears not to be seeing well but who has no physical disease present. The VEP can be particularly useful to estimate the approximate visual acuity in young and multi-disabled children for whom the behavioural methods of assessing acuity may be difficult to perform or interpret. As the pattern of black and white stripes or squares which the child is being shown is gradually reduced in size, the brain signal which is picked up becomes smaller until it becomes undetectable. From this, the approximate visual acuity at a cerebral level can be estimated.

COLOUR VISION AND COLOUR CONTRAST

The most commonly used test for colour vision is the Ishihara colour plate test **(Plate 19)**. Patterns of coloured and grey dots are designed to reveal one pattern to the child with normal colour vision and another to the child with colour confusion. They can be adapted for younger children or those with learning difficulties by getting the child to trace out the pattern with his or her finger rather than naming the figure, or by using plates with pictures instead of numbers. Ishihara plates test only for red-green confusion but other test plates are available for testing blue deficiencies. As mentioned in Chapter 1 this colour vision test was designed to test genetically inherited colour confusions (dichromacy and anomalous colour vision) and may not detect colour deficiencies acquired as a result of retinal or optic nerve disease.

More complex tests include the 100 Hue Test, where the child arranges 84 pastel chips in a colour order which is quite obvious to the child with normal colour vision, but which produces characteristic errors in children with colour confusion. It is quite a difficult test for children to perform and the panel D15 test for children recently developed by Lea Hyvarinen **(Plate 20)**, which involves a smaller number of chips, may be more useful in practice.

CHAPTER 3

DISORDERS OF THE VISUAL SYSTEM AND THEIR IMPLICATIONS

It is important to work with a qualified teacher of visually impaired children to establish the day to day educational implications of a child's visual impairment. The following educational implications described should be used as indicators - all readers should also become familiar with the practical approaches contained in Chapter 4. Where appropriate, children should always be asked what works best for them.

THE FRONT OF THE EYE

a) Congenital abnormalities of the cornea, eg Peter's anomaly, sclerocornea
b) Xerophthalmia
c) Keratoconus
d) Corneal dystrophies
e) Metabolic diseases, eg Hunter's, Hurler's
f) Cataract

a) Congenital abnormalities of the cornea, eg Peter's anomaly (Plate 21), sclerocornea

Definition: Rare disorders of the size or consistency of the cornea which the child is born with.

Cause: The development of the eye structures takes place in early pregnancy and any disturbance which takes place at this time such as maternal illness or the unwitting taking of harmful drugs may cause this and other congenital anomalies. Genetic causes are also possible. Involvement of both eyes is common.

Eye structures affected: The cornea is normally transparent because it is made of very regularly arranged fibres. In sclerocornea, as the name suggests, the fibres of the cornea have taken on the random pattern shown by those of the normal sclera (as opposed to the highly regular lattice structure present in the normal cornea and responsible for its transparency). Hence the whole cornea is white and non-transparent, as though the white of the eye covers the front of the eye. In Peter's anomaly there is usually a central corneal opacity due to a defect in the back layer of the cornea.

Effect on vision: In both cases light cannot get through to the retina and hence there is a profound reduction in visual acuity. It is possible that some useful visual field might remain in an eye where the corneal clouding is only at the centre and some light can get round it to the outer retina. Because this corneal clouding causes severe reduction in vision right from birth, this will tend to cause severe deprivational amblyopia.

Other associations: Associated glaucoma is common in such conditions because the angle between the cornea and iris where aqueous fluid drains out of the eye is also affected. General, non-ocular associations such as learning difficulties are uncommon.

How it is detected: The appearance of the cornea will be abnormal at birth and other causes of corneal opacity (such as those outlined below) must be eliminated by the doctors looking after the baby. This may involve examining the eyes under an anaesthetic as well as general medical investigation.

Medical treatment: The intraocular pressures must be measured (requiring a general anaesthetic in younger children) so that any associated glaucoma can be treated. Surgical management would involve a corneal graft and sometimes in Peter's anomaly removal of the lens and vitreous as well. Corneal grafts are very difficult to manage in young children and even if it were possible, grafting produces a lot of astigmatism which itself produces amblyopia.

One operation which is occasionally helpful involves making a new artificial pupil by cutting a hole in the iris if the normal pupil is covered by a corneal scar - this will at least allow some light into the eye for possible navigational vision. This operation is called an optical iridectomy.

Progression: The corneal opacities are not progressive and indeed in sclerocornea a degree of clearing may occur between the centre and the edge of the cornea. Severe visual impairment is almost inevitable if, as is usual, both eyes are involved.

Educational implications: Both near and distance acuities are severely reduced to variable degrees. The extent of this reduction will determine whether Low Vision Aids (LVAs) will enable print reading or whether braille will be required. Clouding of the cornea can cause uncomfortable glare because of the way light is scattered as it enters the eye. Positioning of light sources and windows behind the child may be both more comfortable for him or her and prevent worsening of visual function (due to scattering of the light by the corneal opacities) if glare is a factor.

b) Vitamin A deficiency and measles (xerophthalmia) (Plate 1)

Definition: Scarring of the cornea due to poor wetting by the tear film caused by vitamin A deficiency.

Cause: In developing countries the diet of children is often deficient in this vitamin. Red meat, liver, green vegetables and carrots are all rich in vitamin A but rice, wheat and maize, often the staple diet in developing countries, are not. Vitamin A is essential for the health of a number of different types of cell in the body including the cells of the conjunctiva, which produce the mucus of the tear film. The health and transparency of the cornea depend on wetting from tears and chronic severe deficiency of this vitamin results in loss of corneal transparency often with blood vessels growing into it. Vitamin A is also a main ingredient for the rod visual pigment, rhodopsin and hence deficiency can also produce night blindness. Another group of cells for which this vitamin is important are the skin cells. After an attack of measles with its accompanying rash, the body's supply of vitamin A is used up as the skin is regenerated. Hence this virus can severely worsen any existing vitamin A deficiency and accelerate the corneal scarring.

From the above explanation it will be clear that this will be a very uncommon cause of visual impairment in developed countries but it remains a very important factor worldwide.

Eye structures affected: Conjunctiva, tear film, cornea and the rod receptors of the retina as above.

Effect on vision: This will depend on the size and position of the corneal scarring, central scars having a more severe effect on visual acuity.

Other associations: These children are often suffering from severe malnutrition and about a quarter will not survive.

How it is detected: Characteristic appearance of the dried-out conjunctiva and cornea in a situation where malnourishment is likely.

Medical treatment: Prevention is by far the most important medical intervention for this condition. This involves education to mothers about diet and, where necessary, supplementary vitamin A given in single large doses. Once the damage has been done medicine or surgery offer little. Corneal grafting is notoriously difficult and gives poor results. An optical iridectomy as explained in the previous section (page 57) may be helpful.

Progression: If severe vitamin A deficiency persists the cornea may thin out and eventually perforate which will cause the eye to collapse and results in permanent and complete blindness in one or both eyes.

Educational implications: These are as explained for the congenital anomalies (page 57) but in the countries where this condition tends to arise, facilities for education of visually impaired children are usually limited if indeed they exist at all. Therefore the outcome may unfortunately be that the child receives no school education.

c) Keratoconus (Plate 22)

Definition: A progressive thinning of the cornea causing it to become cone-shaped.

Cause: There is an association with allergic conjunctivitis which causes itching and it may be that repeated eye rubbing plays a part in causing this condition, but in most cases, no cause is found.

Eye structures affected: The central cornea becomes thinner as the child gets older and becomes the tip of the cone shape

Effect on vision: The distorted shape of the cornea produces astigmatism (page 37). The cornea may lose its transparency in the centre in some cases. Hence visual acuity can be reduced due to distortion and scarring. Educationally significant visual impairment in childhood is rare in the UK.

Other associations: In addition to allergic eye disease, keratoconus is more common in children with Down's syndrome, Marfan's syndrome, retinal dystrophies, aniridia and congenital rubella.

How it is detected: An optician may pick this up by noticing increasing astigmatism, and it may subsequently be confirmed by microscopic examination by the ophthalmologist. In severe cases the conical shape of the cornea can be seen with the naked eye when it is viewed from the side **(Plate 22)**.

Medical treatment: Initially the astigmatism may be managed by spectacles. As the astigmatism progresses, contact lenses may be required. Eventually in the severest cases the cornea becomes so distorted that contact lenses can neither correct it nor stay in the eye. Central corneal scarring (loss of transparency) may also occur. In such cases corneal grafting (see Glossary) will usually be recommended and this is a condition where the outcome of graft surgery is usually very good. Few of these children should therefore nowadays be left with significant visual impairment.

Progression: Mild cases may remain stable and continue to manage with spectacles or contact lenses. In a significant proportion however, as the child progresses through the teens, the distortion and hence the astigmatism worsen and corneal grafting may be considered. There may be short episodes during which the vision worsens severely because the cornea becomes waterlogged - these episodes almost always recover with time and appropriate eyedrop treatment.

Educational implications: This condition is now successfully treated by corneal grafting and few if any affected children require specialist educational input. However keratoconus does sometimes accompany other conditions such as Leber's amaurosis and Down's syndrome and it is therefore worth noting. Children at risk of developing keratoconus should be discouraged from persistent eye rubbing. Visual acuity for near and distance may be reduced by corneal scars or severe astigmatism. Children may require help with contact lens care before or after surgery. Children who do undergo surgery require many hospital visits and the operation should be timed with the child's educational programme in mind. Any child who has undergone a corneal graft should be referred back to the hospital urgently if he or she develops a red eye since there is a risk of the graft rejecting and if a rejection is treated quickly the graft can often be saved.

Footnote: Keratoglobus is a related but much rarer disease involving general thinning of the cornea so that it protrudes in a globular rather than a conical shape. The condition is more difficult to treat than keratoconus and the eyes may perforate after minimal trauma.

d) Corneal Dystrophies

Definition: These are a group of diseases passed on through families and affecting both corneas.

Cause: Genetic

Eye structures affected: Different dystrophies affect different layers of the cornea. For instance congenital hereditary stromal dystrophy (CHSD) affects the middle layer of the cornea, whereas in congenital hereditary endothelial dystrophy (CHED) it is the back layer of the cornea (which usually acts as a pump to keep the cornea dry and hence transparent) which is affected, and so the cornea becomes waterlogged, losing its transparency. Another rare dystrophy called Posterior polymorphous dystrophy (or PPMD) also affects the back layer.

Effect on vision: Although the disease is present from birth, loss of corneal transparency usually progresses with age and only those mentioned above are likely to cause visual impairment in childhood. As for other causes of corneal opacity, visual acuity is reduced and glare may be a problem. Amblyopia may be an additional problem particularly with CHED and PPMD where the cornea is cloudy from birth.

Other associations: None

How it is detected: There may be a family history (though often not in severe cases). Cloudiness of the cornea is noted and microscopic examination of the cornea in the clinic will reveal which layer of the cornea is affected and hence which dystrophy is present.

Medical treatment: Corneal grafting may be required in severe cases though recurrence of the disease in the graft is possible.

Progression: The cornea tends to become more cloudy with time.

Educational implications: The implications of corneal grafting are as for keratoconus (page 59). One of the parents may be affected by the disease in CHED which may help the family understand better the visual difficulties which the child may encounter. As for other conditions with corneal opacity, glare may be a factor. Positioning of the child in the classroom with respect to windows and lights can therefore be important.

e) Metabolic diseases, eg Hunter's syndrome, Hurler's syndrome

Definition: A group of diseases where various compounds are deposited in certain parts of the body (including the cornea) where they should not be.

Cause: The body lacks the ability to digest these particular compounds.

Eye structures affected: Cornea, retina and optic nerve to varying degrees. Glaucoma may also be present.

Effect on vision: This depends on which of the above parts of the eye are worst affected. If the cornea is the main problem the effect on vision will be as for the corneal dystrophies; if it is the retina it will be as for retinitis pigmentosa, and if it is the optic nerve then the effects will be as for optic atrophy.

Other associations: These may include learning difficulties, deafness and abnormalities of facial appearance and skeletal structure. Life expectancy may be significantly shortened.

How it is detected: From the combinations of the above features and biochemical tests.

Medical treatment: Paediatricians will be involved in the general medical care of the child. Corneal grafting is sometimes performed but often the additional retinal or optic nerve damage or severe learning difficulties make it unhelpful.

Progression: The retinopathy and glaucoma may be progressive.

Educational implications: The child will be facing multiple problems. The educational implications of corneal disease, retinal dystrophy and optic atrophy may all need to be considered in addition to possible hearing impairment and learning difficulties.

f) Cataract (Plates 23-24)

Definition: Loss of transparency of the lens as shown in **Plate 23.**

Cause: A variety of causes include genetic, infections affecting the mother during pregnancy, general biochemical disorders of childhood which affect the eye (such as defects in the way certain sugars or calcium salts are handled). Sometimes no cause is found.

Eye structures affected: By definition it is the lens of the eye which is affected. Sometimes cataract may be part of a syndrome affecting other parts of the eye as well: for example, aniridia and microphthalmos.

Effect on vision: It has recently been discovered that good vision during the first three months of life is critical for the growth and development of the visual brain. When cataracts are discovered at birth, cataract surgery is ideally carried out during the first few weeks of life (provided the cataracts are severe enough to be significantly affecting vision) and replacement lenses given straight away. In cases where surgery has been delayed there may be permanent significant visual impairment (called deprivational amblyopia) despite later surgery, because the initial programming of the visual brain has not taken place. Children born with cataract in one eye rarely regain useful vision following surgery in the affected eye since deprivation amblyopia is exaggerated when the other eye sees well, although such children will not be visually impaired.

Some opacities of the lens are of no consequence and may not even be noticed. The effect on vision depends on:

a) The age of onset – cataracts present at birth or in infancy can cause severe amblyopia;

b) The density of the opacity - ie how much light can pass through it and;

c) Position – opacities in the centre of the lens interrupt light passing to the macula and therefore tend to cause a more severe loss of acuity than opacities situated near the edge of the lens.

In addition to reduction in vision, cataracts can cause light entering the eye to be scattered therefore causing the child to experience glare. This is particularly common if the opacity is situated towards the back of the lens, and this type of cataract is often associated with retinitis pigmentosa and uveitis.

Other associations: Cataract may be associated with a variety of disorders affecting the eye such as the rubella syndrome, retinitis pigmentosa, chronic uveitis, aniridia and many others. It may also be associated with disorders affecting the rest of the body such as Down's syndrome, or the biochemical disorders mentioned above.

How it is detected: Since early treatment is very important for successful treatment of cataracts present at birth, it is essential that they are detected very soon after birth. Doctors in charge of babies make a routine examination of the whole baby soon after birth and this should include shining an ophthalmoscope at the eye and looking at the pupil which normally has a reddish glow (as seen in flash photography). Significant cataract will block this 'red reflex' showing as a black shadow **(Plate 23)**. Thus all newborn babies are 'screened' for cataract. Suspicious cases are then referred to an ophthalmologist for examination with the microscope.

Medical treatment: Children with cataracts significantly affecting the vision of both eyes require cataract surgery which involves removing the lenses. Absence of the lens is termed aphakia. The lens accounts for about a third of the eye's refractive power and its absence results in reduced focusing power. All aphakic people used to have to wear thick, convex spectacle lenses **(Plate 24)** after cataract surgery to correct this, but now almost all adults undergoing cataract surgery have an artificial lens implant inserted in the same site as the natural lens. This removes the need for such thick glasses and gives much less distortion of images than the glasses used to. There is an increasing trend towards the insertion of such implants in infants and children as well, but there are a number of technical problems associated with this so it has not been popular in the recent past. There are a large number of school-age children at present who have had cataracts removed and have not had artificial lenses implanted. They require either contact lenses or thick glasses (called aphakic glasses) to achieve a clear image. Contact lenses give a better quality of image and may therefore be preferable if they can be tolerated by the child and managed by the family. Indeed, aphakic spectacles enlarge the image so much (a side effect of their thickness) that they cannot be used unless both eyes are aphakic, since if one eye is normal, the sizes of the images created by the two eyes would be so different that the brain could not combine them resulting in double vision. Whichever form of optical correction is used (including the intra-ocular lens implant), extra reading glasses are essential for near work since, as described in Chapter 1, it is the elasticity of the natural lens which allows the eye to focus on near objects (accommodation) and this variable focus is absent in aphakia.

The trend is towards early surgery if it is required. The other trend is towards implanting artificial lenses wherever possible even in very young babies. It is of course essential that aphakic children (especially under the age of eight) wear their aphakic optical correction all the time, be it glasses or contact lenses, because, as we have said, blurred images in young children can lead to permanent amblyopia. Even if a lens implant is present, glasses or contact lenses may also be necessary since as the eye grows, its focusing power changes. Reading glasses will certainly be required before school is started because the lens implants in current use do not have the facility to change shape as the natural *'elastic'* lens does to bring the normal eye into focus (Chapter 1). Usually further surgical or laser procedures are required if the lens capsule (left in place at the initial operation to support the lens implant) thickens up causing a similar blurring of vision to the initial cataract.

Progression: This is variable. Some cataracts may not interfere with vision when first detected, but the child needs to be watched carefully over time in case vision gets worse and requires surgery at a later stage. Other cataracts may never progress to a stage requiring surgery.

Educational implications: Children should be encouraged to wear their glasses or contact lenses at all times at home and school. Separate reading glasses will usually be required for close work. Bright diffuse lighting without glare will improve visual performance in many cases. This is because it causes the pupil to become smaller, resulting in greater depth of focus, allowing the child to see more clearly for near, distance and intermediate distances (see page 12). The teacher should look out for any apparent deterioration in vision in the child with unoperated cataract (where the cataract may be getting worse) or with operated cataract (where capsule thickening may occur as explained above). Frequent hospital visits and sometimes multiple operations may be necessary which may interfere with school, and should ideally be planned during school holidays if practicable and appropriate.

THE WHOLE EYE

a)   Infections passed from mother to child during pregnancy
b)   Absent or very small eyes
c)   Coloboma (plural - colobomata) **(Plate 25)**
d)   Albinism **(Plate 26)**
e)   Aniridia **(Plate 28)**
f)   Childhood glaucoma **(Plate 29)**

a) Infections passed from mother to child during pregnancy

Definition: Most infections acquired during pregnancy do not damage the developing foetus but there are some notable exceptions, including those listed.

Cause: During pregnancy, virus infections such as rubella, cytomegalovirus (CMV), and the AIDS virus (HIV) as well as other types of infection such as toxoplasma and syphilis may damage the foetus and the developing visual system. The incidence of rubella has decreased dramatically with the widespread introduction of effective vaccination, but the incidence of HIV infection is on the increase.

Toxoplasma infection is acquired from eating undercooked meat or by eating unwashed vegetables contaminated by infected cat faeces. It is the most common infective cause of childhood visual impairment in developed countries, but fortunately only affects one eye in most cases.

Eye structures affected: Almost any part of the eye can be affected but there are certain characteristic features. Rubella infection causes greatest damage to the foetus during the first three months of pregnancy when the organs such as the eye, ear and heart are being formed. Because of this the eye may be underdeveloped and smaller than it should be (microphthalmos). Other ocular features of the rubella syndrome include congenital cataract (the clouding is usually in the centre of the lens and will significantly reduce acuity and require early surgery to prevent amblyopia); a mottling of the retina (pigmentary retinopathy) which may progress with age but usually only reduces the acuity to around 6/12 if no other parts of the eye are affected; corneal clouding and glaucoma (usually associated with microphthalmos).

Foetal damage in general, and ocular involvement in particular, are less common after CMV infection but can include, in addition to the above, inflammation of the choroid and retina (chorioretinitis) and damage to the optic nerve (optic atrophy).

Life expectancy for children infected with HIV has been poor but as treatment improves these children may live long enough for visual impairment to become a concern – certainly HIV infected adults may become severely visually impaired usually fairly near the end of the course of this fatal disease. The cause is a viral infection of the retina (usually CMV) and this is an example of the reduced immune defences of the body allowing a virus, which rarely has serious consequences in a person with normal immune defences, to cause serious damage to the AIDS patient.

The damage from toxoplasma infection usually also involves inflammation in the retina and choroid. This may be present at birth but there are examples of infected infants being apparently normal at initial examination who develop severe visual impairment even years later. Microphthalmos, cataract and optic atrophy can also occur. Syphilis is, like rubella, now uncommon in the UK, though it is seen more frequently in some other countries. Corneal clouding is the best known manifestation of congenital syphilis but all the other defects mentioned above with other infections can occur.

Effect on vision: Microphthalmos is usually associated with poor vision making associated cataract and glaucoma difficult to treat. Cataract and corneal clouding tend to cause reduction in visual acuity as does chorioretinitis affecting the macula. Peripheral retinal inflammation, optic atrophy and glaucoma may all cause additional loss of visual field.

Other associations: The following features are particularly associated but the list is not exhaustive. Neither are these features always present:

- Rubella: growth retardation, congenital heart defects (such as a hole in the heart), auditory impairment.
- CMV: malformations of the brain with associated learning and motor disorders.
- HIV: prone to a number of disabling and dangerous infections and tumours; reduced life expectancy.

- Toxoplasma: calcium deposition in the brain, epilepsy, hydrocephalus.
- Syphilis: auditory impairment, teeth malformations, bone malformations.

How it is detected: The mother may be aware of an infection (eg rubella) during pregnancy but quite often there may be no such history. Toxoplasma and CMV infections, for instance, often pass unnoticed in adults. Blood tests can be performed (in mother and child) to measure antibody levels to specific infections if they are suspected - if antibody levels are raised, this indicates recent infection and helps make the diagnosis.

Medical treatment: Cataract surgery may be indicated and corneal grafting is occasionally helpful. Inflammation may recur in the older child (eg toxoplasma in the retina) and this may require treatment with antibiotic and steroid tablets. Therefore if a pupil with a known diagnosis of toxoplasmosis complains of a recent deterioration or distortion of vision then an urgent referral to the ophthalmology clinic is appropriate since drugs may damp down the inflammation and help preserve remaining vision.

Progression: Although the damage in these conditions is present at birth, sometimes the infecting organism stays in the body and the eye of the child for years and can cause progressive damage or recurrent attacks of inflammation. If glaucoma is present this can cause progressive visual field loss. As is always the case with significant cataract or corneal clouding present at birth, the potential for severe deprivational amblyopia exists if the vision is not surgically cleared quickly.

Educational implications: These are very variable depending on which parts of the eyes are affected in a particular child and which non-ocular abnormalities are also present.

b) Absent or very small eyes

Definition: A range of abnormalities of development of the eye including complete failure of development with no eye present (anophthalmos); incomplete development and a small eye (microphthalmos); small eyes with varying degrees of skin covering them (cryptophthalmos).

Cause: These are usually *'one-off'* anomalies rather than being passed on in families. A number of environmental factors have been implicated including maternal infection during pregnancy, radiation, and chemical exposure. There are also some genetic syndromes which include anophthalmos or microphthalmos as part of a wide range of abnormalities. In most cases no specific cause is identified.

Eye structures affected: In microphthalmos the cornea is usually but not always small. The pupil may be an odd shape due to coloboma of the iris. This condition is dealt with in more detail in section c but represents a failure of a cleft in the developing eye of the embryo to close properly.

Effect on vision: In bilateral anophthalmos blindness is inevitable. In microphthalmos the degree of visual impairment depends on the severity of the abnormality in each eye.

Other associations: There are a number of syndromes which include microphthalmos for example the CHARGE syndrome which comprises heart defects, nasal abnormalities, growth retardation, genital and ear anomalies.

How it is detected: The defect is often obvious on examination though careful examination or even ultrasound or X-ray scanning may be required to detect buried remnants of poorly developed eyes.

Medical treatment: The level of vision must be ascertained and any refractive error corrected (small eyes are likely to be long sighted (hypermetropic)). Long sighted spectacle lenses will also make the eye appear bigger to others and may therefore provide a cosmetic improvement (long sighted lenses always have a magnifying effect). Cosmetic contact lenses or shells may be appropriate for non-seeing eyes. Glaucoma may be associated and this must be treated with surgery and or eye drops.

Progression: These developmental abnormalities are likely to be non-progressive. Associated glaucoma may however cause progressive visual field loss.

Educational implications: Visual impairment may be severe, microphthalmos accounting for 10% of blind children in one study. Braille usage may be required.

c) **Coloboma (plural - colobomata) (Plate 25)**

Definition: A notch-like defect in any part or parts of the eye from the eyelid at the front to the optic nerve or retina at the back which is present at birth and is non-progressive.

Cause: Any interference with the development of the eye in the embryo can cause a coloboma. The notch-like cleft is present in the developing eye and the normal process is for the two edges of the cleft to grow towards each other and then join. It is failure of this joining which results in the coloboma. Rarely the cause can be genetic. Often, as for many other congenital anomalies, no cause is found.

Eye structures affected: Any eye structure can be affected, the eyelid, iris, lens, optic disc and retina being among the more common. The size of the defect varies from being barely noticeable to an almost complete absence of the structure involved. Optic disc and retinal colobomata may result in retinal detachment later in life.

Effect on vision: This will depend on the size and the position of the defect. In general, larger defects and those nearer the back of the eye (optic disc and retina) are more likely to cause visual impairment. There may be other associated abnormalities within the eyes, or occasionally within the visual pathways of the brain, which may affect vision.

Other associations: A large number of associated conditions can occur both within and outside the eye. Colobomata affecting both eyes may be associated with some abnormalities of the central part of the brain which is responsible both for control of hormones (for example growth and sexual development) and for the connections between the right and left sides of the brain.

Microphthalmos or anophthalmos can be thought of as the most extreme type of colobomata and in some genetic cases both microphthalmos and colobomata may be present in different eyes of different family members.

One relatively common syndrome associated with optic nerve colobomata may result in dual sensory impairment (other causes including congenital rubella and Usher's disease) and has acquired the mnemonic CHARGE syndrome, representing Coloboma, Heart defect, Atresia (narrowing) of the nostrils, Retardation of growth (and sometimes intellectual development), Genital anomalies and Ear abnormalities and deafness.

How it is detected: Colobomata affecting the front structures of the eyes (eg the lid or iris) are easily noticeable. Smaller, more subtle defects and those at the back of the eyes are detected by ophthalmological examination.

Medical treatment: Surgery is rarely useful but may be so if there is a large defect in the eyelid resulting in exposure of the front of the eye or if there is an associated retinal detachment. Any associated ocular or non-ocular conditions must be treated appropriately.

Progression: The defect itself is non-progressive although, as explained, complications may develop progressively such as damage to the cornea because it is not adequately covered, or retinal detachment.

Educational implications: These are as variable as the condition itself. Only children with both eyes affected may be visually impaired. Severe anomalies may produce significant visual and cosmetic impairment. Large iris colobomata may result in photophobia and reduced vision in bright focal lighting conditions similar to that experienced by children with aniridia. The importance of specialised training for the teachers of children with dual sensory impairment (whether due to CHARGE syndrome, Usher's syndrome or other causes) is well-recognised.

d) Albinism (Plate 26)

Definition: Any congenital condition in which the colouration (pigmentation) is reduced involving the skin and the eyes (oculocutaneous albinism), or the eyes alone (ocular albinism).

Cause: This is a genetic condition, though the way it is inherited varies. Some forms are passed down through the generations (dominant), some occur with no warning when both parents are coincidental carriers without the disease (recessive) and some forms affect only male children but are passed on only through female carriers (X or sex linked). The more severe forms tend to have recessive inheritance and the milder forms dominant. Albinism affecting only the eyes (ocular albinism) tends to be inherited as X-linked. (See Glossary for more details of these inheritance types.)

Eye structures affected: The iris and choroid lack coloration and in obvious cases the light reflected from the retina through the iris may give the eye a reddish appearance. The fovea is not properly developed and there is some miswiring of nerve fibres where they cross.

Effect on vision: The abnormal fovea means that visual acuity is reduced and this is associated with nystagmus (or wobbly eyes). (Other diseases which cause severe visual impairment from birth, such as untreated cataract or cone dystrophy, may also be associated with nystagmus.) Distance vision tends to be more affected than near, probably because the nystagmus is less for near vision **(Plate 8)** and hence the image is stabilised. The degree of visual impairment can vary with visual acuities between 6/9 and 6/60 in the majority of cases. The lack of coloration in the iris and choroid means that too much light enters the eye and is not absorbed properly. Therefore bright light causes discomfort which is called photophobia. In focal bright light conditions the image can be degraded **(Plate 27)**. Refractive errors and squint are common.

Other associations: Children with oculocutaneous albinism lack colouration in the skin as well as the eye. This coloration is protective against the harmful effects of sunlight and hence these children are more prone to skin cancers. Appropriate skin care is therefore required. This is a more significant risk in hot countries where the normal population have darker skin for greater protection from the sun. In such countries light skinned people with albinism will also look more noticeably different from the normal population and may suffer correspondingly more social stigma. Rarer associations include repeated infections (Chediak Higashi syndrome) and easy bruisability (Hermansky-Pudlak syndrome). There is some evidence that people with oculocutaneous albinism have a tendency to have a high IQ.

How it is detected: Ophthalmic examination may reveal subtle thinning of the iris in mild cases as well as light coloration of the choroid. Nystagmus may be the first indication, and knowledge that other family members are affected, or examination of family members to detect subtle disease or gene carriers may be helpful.

Medical treatment: Any refractive errors must be corrected and low vision aids are often helpful. Tinted lenses are helpful in reducing photophobia.

Progression: The disease is non-progressive.

Educational implications: Positioning in the classroom is important both in relation to lighting (having windows and lights behind the child rather than in front will reduce photophobia as will the use of translucent material to diffuse the sunlight) and in relation to distance from the blackboard, remembering that distance vision is usually poorer than near.

e) Aniridia (Plate 28)

Definition: This is a group of disorders involving under-development of the iris.

Cause: This is caused by an error in the genes (mutation), sometimes passed on from parents and sometimes arising as a new mutation.

Eye structures affected: Almost all the eye structures can be affected. Although the iris may appear to be completely absent to the naked eye there is usually a microscopically small stump of iris present. Corneal opacities, cataract, lens dislocation, glaucoma and optic nerve hypoplasia can be present in varying combinations in some cases.

Effect on vision: Glare and photophobia are problems due to the lack of protection of the eye from light by the iris. The acuity may be reduced due to any of the above features or combinations of them.

Other associations: This condition can be associated with the kidney tumour called Wilm's tumour though this is uncommon in the inherited form. Other abnormalities of the kidneys, learning difficulties and growth retardation have also all been associated.

How it is detected: The characteristic reddish appearance of the eye results from the absence of iris tissue.

Medical treatment: This involves correction of any refractive errors which might be present and provision of tinted glasses to reduce the amount of light getting into the eye. Occluder contact lenses with an artificial iris painted on have also been tried for this purpose. Cataract and glaucoma may require surgical treatment.

Progression: Corneal problems and glaucoma may follow in later life.

Educational implications: Positioning of the child in the classroom needs consideration with light sources behind him or her. As for albinism, diffuse lighting is preferable to focal lighting. LVAs may be appropriate when acuities are reduced. The child may be concerned about the unusual appearance of the eyes in which case cosmetic contact lenses may be helpful. Regular hospital visits may be necessary if glaucoma or cataract are present.

f) Childhood glaucoma (Plate 29)

Definition: A range of conditions all involving the pressure inside the eye being too high and causing progressive damage to the optic nerve and impairing vision.

Cause: The exact cause of straightforward childhood glaucoma is not known though hereditary factors are thought to play a part.

Eye structures affected: The wall of the young eye (sclera and cornea) is more elastic than that of the adult eye and it will stretch when the pressure inside it goes up, enlarging the eye (buphthalmos) mentioned earlier. The stretching of the cornea may damage its transparency and leave characteristic stretch marks, visible under high magnification. As explained in Chapter 1, the optic disc where the optic nerve leaves the eye is vulnerable to damage by raised pressure and the nerve fibres can progressively die and disappear as they pass through the disc.

Effect on vision: In many cases early detection and surgical treatment controls the pressure and prevents loss of vision, but blindness can occur in a minority of cases. Corneal stretching, damage to the optic nerve and amblyopia due to visual deprivation at an early age all contribute to the visual impairment. Optic nerve damage at the optic disc usually affects parts of the peripheral field of vision before central visual acuity is lost because nerve fibres from the peripheral retina are the most susceptible to raised pressure.

Other associations: Glaucoma can also occur as a part of or as a result of several other conditions affecting the eye such as aniridia, rubella syndrome, Reiger's anomaly (a group of conditions running in families in which the pupil may be an irregular shape and the iris is abnormal), uveitis (particularly the type of uveitis associated with childhood arthritis) and retinopathy of prematurity.

How it is detected: Apart from enlargement of the eye and corneal clouding which may be obvious, affected infants characteristically rub their eyes and may dislike bright light. The eyes will often water a lot (though glaucoma is an extremely rare cause of watery eyes in infancy).

Medical treatment: Surgery is usually required to achieve a lasting reduction in pressure though even if this is achieved, a significant proportion of eyes may remain visually impaired. Because the eye may be enlarged, a refractive error is likely to be present (enlargement of the eye tends to cause myopia as explained in Chapter 2) and prescription of appropriate glasses may help the child make full use of available vision. Eye drop treatment to maintain a low pressure in the eye may be required in the long term.

Progression: Once the pressure in the eye is controlled the visual impairment should not progress. Uncontrolled pressure will result in progressive damage to the optic nerve and with it the visual field.

Educational implications: Visual impairment may involve acuity (corneal clouding and amblyopia) and/or peripheral visual field (optic disc damage). Both factors must be considered for each child, remembering that children with limited acuity may benefit from sitting close to the front of a class and possibly from LVAs, and that children with limited peripheral vision may have only partial visual appreciation of the classroom environment around them and may need help with mobility. Classroom lighting needs to be considered since photophobia can be a feature, in which

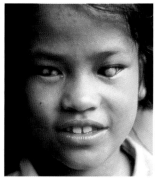

Plate 1 Cosmetically noticeable and visual impairing corneal scars of both eyes caused by Vitamin A deficiency

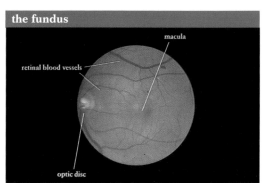

Plate 2 Fundus

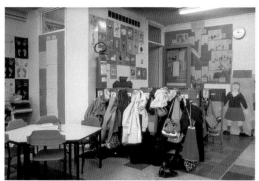

Plate 3 Colour confusion

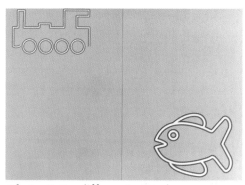

Plate 4 Cardiff acuity cards

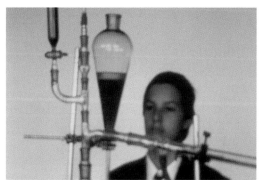

Plate 5 View with a visual acuity of 6/18

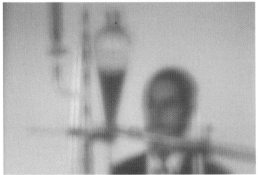

Plate 6 Blurred focus due to uncorrected refractive error

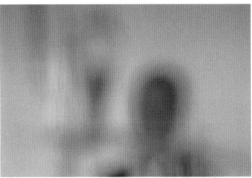

Plate 7 Reduced visual acuity (3/60)

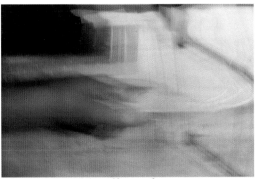

Plate 8 Possible effect of nystagmus on vision

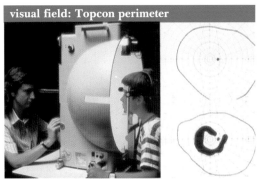

Plate 9 Topcon perimeter

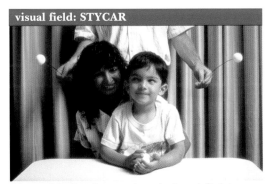

Plate 10 Confrontational visual field testing

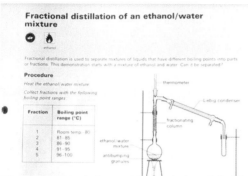

Plate 11 Worksheet: Normal visual field

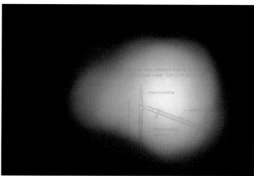

Plate 12 Worksheet: Peripheral visual field loss

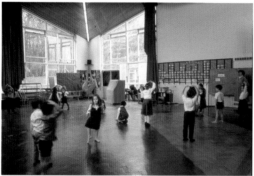

Plate 13 Hall: Normal visual field

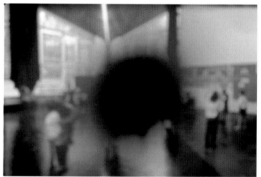

Plate 14 Hall: Central visual field loss

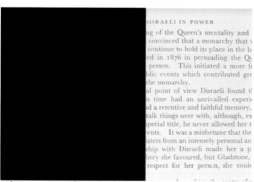

Plate 15 Left sided visual loss (homonymous hemianopia)

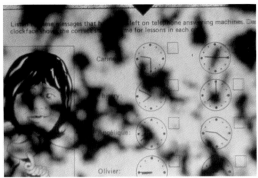

Plate 16 Interrupted visual field

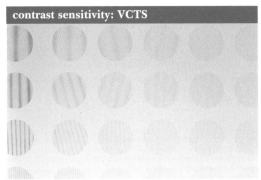

Plate 17 Contrast sensitivity test

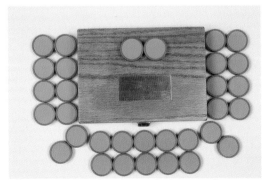

Plate 18 Electroretinography (ERG) testing using skin electrodes

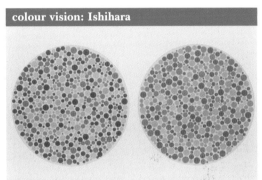

Plate 19 Ishihara test

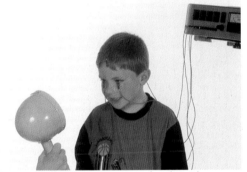

Plate 20 Pastel coloured chips to be arranged by child as developed by Lea Hyvarinen

81

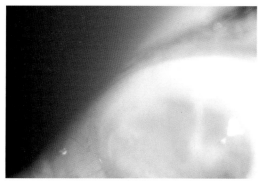

Plate 21 Congenital abnormality of the cornea

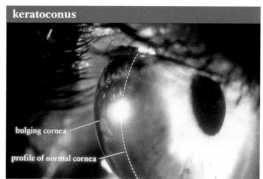

Plate 22 Keratoconus

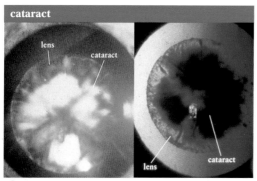

Plate 23 Cataract

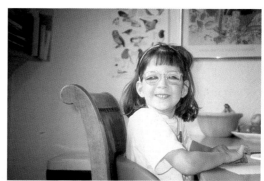

Plate 24 Aphakic spectacles

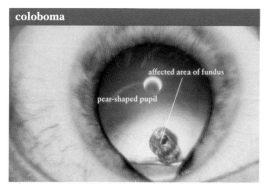

Plate 25 Coloboma

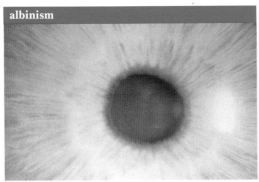

Plate 26 Albinism

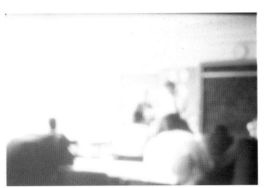

Plate 27 Photophobia

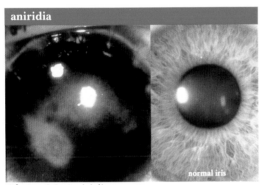

Plate 28 Aniridia

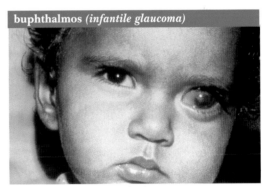

Plate 29 Childhood glaucoma (buphthalmos)

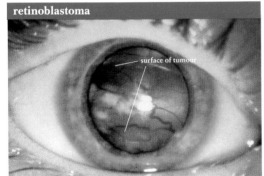

Plate 30 Retinoblastoma

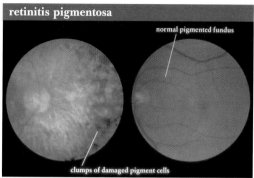

Plate 31 Retinitis pigmentosa

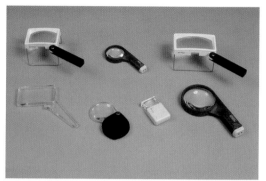

Plate 32 Hand-held LVAs

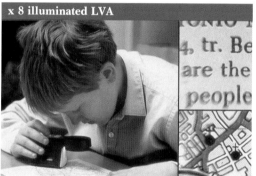

Plate 33 x8 illuminated LVA

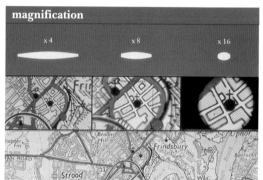

Plate 34 Magnification of maps

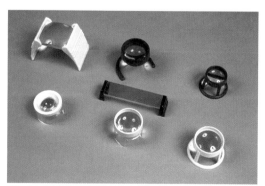

Plate 35 Stand magnifiers

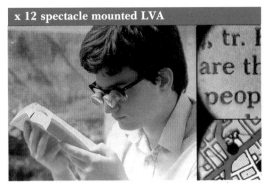

Plate 36 Spectacle mounted magnifier

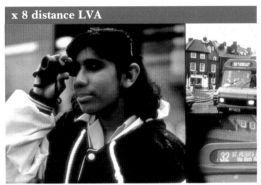

Plate 37 Telescopic systems

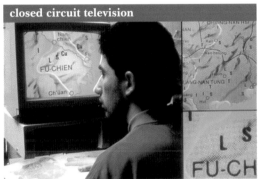

Plate 38 Closed circuit TVs (CCTVs)

case diffuse lighting is therefore preferable. The wearing of glasses if appropriate should be encouraged. The child may be self-conscious about the unusual appearance of the eyes which may be different sizes from each other or obviously enlarged. Regular hospital visits and repeat operations are sometimes necessary which may interfere with schooling.

THE BACK OF THE EYE

a) Retinoblastoma **(Plate 30)**
b) Retinopathy of prematurity
c) Stationary night blindness
d) Stationary cone disorders
e) Leber's amaurosis
f) Retinitis pigmentosa **(Plate 31)**
g) Macular dystrophies
h) Norrie's disease and Incontinenta pigmenta
i) Batten's disease

a) Retinoblastoma (Plate 30)

Definition: This is the commonest cancer of the eye which occurs in childhood. It consists of a tumour or tumours of retinal cells and usually develops before the age of four.

Cause: The cause of this disease is an abnormality in a particular gene responsible for normal cell growth in the retina. This mutation predisposes to tumour formation and may be passed down the generations of a family in the inherited type of the disease. Isolated cases can also occur in which the mutation has taken place in a single cell in the retina. Genetic testing can reveal whether a child who survives retinoblastoma but has not inherited it from the family (an isolated case) is at risk of passing the disease on to his or her children.

Eye structures affected: The tumour(s) arise(s) in the retina but can spread forward into the rest of the eye or backward along the optic nerve. Inherited retinoblastoma is more likely to produce multiple tumours and to affect both eyes than the non-hereditary form. The inherited disease tends to arise in younger children than the non-hereditary form.

Effect on vision: Children with only one eye affected may not be visually impaired, but if both eyes are involved, one eye may have been removed surgically and the vision of the surviving eye depends on the size and position of the original retinal tumour. Small tumours well away from the macula may have little effect on vision, whereas those involving the macula may significantly impair vision even if the tumour itself responds well to treatment.

Other associations: This is a potentially fatal condition and if untreated death is almost inevitable. With modern treatment, however, more than 90% of children survive.

How it is detected: The tumour is usually picked up because the pupil appears white rather than the normal black appearance. A squint or a red painful eye are alternative presentations. All children with a family history should be examined regularly and the disorder detected at an early stage. Examination by an ophthalmologist reveals white tumours in the retina in one or both eyes. Scanning of the brain or other organs such as the liver may be necessary to see if the cancer has spread, so that appropriate treatment can be planned.

Medical treatment: The medical care in retinoblastoma involves careful examination and investigation of the child for any sign that the cancer might be spreading. Treatment of the tumour itself may involve removal of the whole eye (enucleation) when the other eye is healthy and unaffected. If both eyes are affected the worse affected eye may be removed or treated with radiation and the tumour in the better eye may be treated with radiation, freezing or laser. Anti-cancer drugs may also form part of the treatment. Only occasionally is removal of both eyes necessary. Genetic counselling is offered to the family members, particularly about the complicated genetics and the risks to other and future family members.

Progression: New retinal tumours or recurrences of treated ones are most likely in the first year after diagnosis.

Educational implications: The type and severity of visual impairment depends on whether both eyes are involved, where the tumours are situated in the retina and how big they are. For example, tumours involving the macula are likely to have a severe effect on acuity and central vision. Radiotherapy may sometimes cause cataract development which poses a further threat to vision. In addition to visual impairment there are the psychological implications of a child having to cope with cancer and possible removal of an eye. These psychological effects may be influenced in hereditary cases by the previous experiences of other family members. Because of the complexity of medical treatment and the risks of recurrence, regular hospital visits, some prolonged, are inevitable; such visits may be sight and life-saving but may severely interfere with education and, if practicable, should be timed as far as is possible in conjunction with educational needs and programmes in mind.

b) Retinopathy of prematurity

Definition: A scarring disease of the retina developing in premature and low birth-weight infants. The disease used to be known as retrolental fibroplasia.

Cause: This disease has developed only relatively recently (1942) as the care and therefore survival of severely premature babies has dramatically improved. Before this, babies at risk of the condition would not have survived. Retinopathy of prematurity is becoming an increasingly common cause of visual impairment in developing countries as the quality and availability of neonatal care improves.

The exact cause of the condition is not known, but relates to the fact that the blood vessels which supply the retina are not fully developed until a baby reaches full term, and so when babies are born very prematurely, parts of the retina do not have adequate blood supply. In the early cases, excessive oxygen therapy was thought to be the principal cause, but now this is administered to babies at risk more cautiously. This has resulted in a reduction in the frequency of the disease but not eradication, and it is likely that other factors relating to birth weight and genetics also play a part.

Eye structures affected: The retina is the main site of the problem and there are various stages of severity of involvement. The milder degrees of the disorder usually resolve spontaneously and only the more severe stages require any form of treatment. These severe stages involve scarring of the retina and most severe of all, the retina being pulled away from its normal position against the choroid (retinal detachment). As explained in Chapter 1, the retina depends on the choroid for most of its oxygen supply, and therefore such detachment from the choroid produces permanent damage to the retina.

Other effects on the eye seen in this condition include myopic refractive errors, squint (misalignment of the eyes so that they are not looking in the same direction), amblyopia and optic atrophy.

Effect on vision: As understanding of the condition and its prevention and treatment has increased, the outlook for vision has improved significantly, so that serious eye disease is now largely confined to infants of less than 1000g birthweight. Even among these children, only a minority become blind in both eyes. In less affected children, acuity may be reduced by macular scarring, amblyopia or optic atrophy, and the peripheral visual field may be affected by peripheral retinal scarring or optic atrophy.

Other associations: Because these children are usually born prematurely there is a relatively high incidence of associated brain damage, which may cause learning difficulties and cerebral palsy.

How it is detected: Currently all premature and low birthweight babies at risk should be examined by an ophthalmologist so that any disease requiring treatment can be detected.

Medical treatment: This is performed either with a freezing probe applied to the outside of the eye which freezes right through the wall of the eye onto the affected retina, or with a laser beam directed at the affected retina through the pupil. If severe scarring and detachment develop, complex surgery is occasionally carried out, but the results of this are often very disappointing in terms of the vision achieved. Older children may require patching therapy for amblyopia, and refraction and correction of the short sightedness which commonly accompanies the disease.

Progression: The disease develops and progresses only during the first weeks of life and it is during this time that careful examination is required. Once the child reaches school age, any damage will have been done and further progression would not be expected.

Educational implications: These of course vary with the severity of the visual impairment which varies from mild to blindness, indicating possible braille usage. The macula is often involved and Low Vision Aids (LVAs) may therefore be helpful in addition to spectacles for myopia. Additional learning or movement control disorders (cerebral palsy) may be present, posing additional challenges to the child, family and teachers.

c) Stationary night blindness

Definition: This is a non-progressive inherited retinal dystrophy in which difficulty seeing in the dark is the principal feature.

Cause: This is genetic and it may be inherited in a dominant, recessive or sex-linked form.

Eye structures affected: The rods and cones of the retina are abnormal, although the retina looks normal when it is examined. Other features which may be associated are marked short sightedness (high myopia), nystagmus or squint.

Effect on vision: Difficulty seeing in the dark is the main effect but some children, particularly with the recessive or sex-linked forms of the disease may have reduced acuity (these children are more likely to have nystagmus).

Other associations: Two other forms of stationary night blindness are called Oguchi's disease and fundus albipunctatus, but these do not normally cause a reduction in visual acuity and there may not therefore be special educational needs.

How it is detected: The complaints of difficulty seeing in the dark associated with poor vision and a normal looking retina will lead to electrical tests being performed as explained in Chapter 2 (p.51) and these have a characteristic appearance in this disorder.

Medical treatment: No treatment is available for the actual disorder of the retinal receptors, but associated problems such as myopia and squint can be treated.

Progression: By definition this disease is not progressive.

Educational implications: Good levels of lighting will help the child maximise vision. For children with reduced acuities, LVAs may be helpful.

d) Stationary cone disorders (achromatopsia)

Definition: These are non-progressive retinal disorders affecting visual acuity and colour vision.

Cause: Genetic, inherited in recessive or sex-linked forms.

Eye structures affected: As the name suggests it is the cone receptors which are affected and may be completely absent (known as rod monochromatism) or in less severe types only the blue cones are present (blue cone monochromatism), the red and green cones being absent. High hypermetropia, nystagmus and photophobia may be present.

Effect on vision: The vision is often better in dim illumination. The visual acuity is about 6/60 with absent colour vision in the most severe form in which the cones are completely absent (called rod monochromatism). Less severe forms may have better acuities. Peripheral visual fields are usually intact, though there may be a defect (or scotoma) in the central field. This is because peripheral vision is mediated by rods and cones whereas central vision and acuity are mediated by cones only (Chapter 1).

Other associations: None is known.

How it is detected: A combination of the above features and abnormal electrical tests give the diagnosis. As explained in Chapter 2, the electrical tests can be used to distinguish between faulty cone function such as in this condition, and faulty rod function which is a major feature of retinitis pigmentosa.

Medical treatment: As for other retinal dystrophies, there is no specific medical treatment available but associated refractive errors must be looked for and treated.

Progression: By definition these conditions are non-progressive.

Educational implications: The main limitations to be borne in mind in the provision of material are reduced acuity and reduced or absent colour vision. LVAs and or large print may therefore be beneficial. Dim lighting conditions will often help the child. Tinted glasses and sometimes dark goggles may also be used to produce darkened conditions with associated improved vision.

NB A related condition called cone-rod dystrophy or cone dystrophy tends to present later in adults or older children with decreased vision and photophobia. Visual acuity gradually deteriorates to 6/60 and later involvement of rods is also common, giving similar symptoms to retinitis pigmentosa (page 95).

e) Leber's amaurosis

Definition: An inherited retinal dystrophy (dystrophy means an inherited weakness or disorder) involving both rod and cone receptors and causing problems from birth or the first few months of life. Amaurosis comes from the Latin meaning blindness.

Cause: This is genetic and is inherited in a recessive way. This means that both parents are coincidentally carriers of the disease without suffering from the disease and are unaware of the fact that they are carriers until one of their children is affected - each child that they have has a one in four risk of being affected by the disease, and children without the disease have a two in three risk of being a carrier.

Eye structures affected: Although the retina may look normal to the examining ophthalmologist in the early stages, most children develop the characteristic features of a retinal dystrophy as they get older. These include a black speckling on the retina, narrowing of the retinal arteries and the optic disc becoming pale. The eyes do not lock onto targets in the normal way because vision is poor from birth or a very young age, and roving eye movements and nystagmus result. The child may poke his or her eyes since mechanical stimulation of the retina can send signals up the visual pathway which are perceived as flashes of light. Children often have high hypermetropic or occasionally high myopic refractive errors. Cataract and keratoconus may develop in older children and in some cases may be due to habitual eye rubbing.

Effect on vision: Both peripheral visual field and visual acuity are severely affected in this condition because both rods and cones are affected. Visual acuities tend to range from 3/60 to perception of light. It is a relatively common cause of blindness in children.

Other associations: Most cases of Leber's amaurosis occur in otherwise normal children. However a variety of associated problems including learning difficulties, and a range of brain disorders, as well as kidney and heart problems can occur. The frequency with which brain disorders are reported has decreased in recent years and this is due in part to the recognition of specific syndromes involving the retina and brain (see next section) which might have previously been wrongly ascribed a diagnosis of Leber's amaurosis. Moreover, the recognition that blind children may reach some developmental milestones later than sighted children and that this is not due to additional brain damage but simply to blindness has led to fewer cases of 'brain damage' being reported. Hearing difficulties occur in about 5% of children with Leber's amaurosis.

How it is detected: The combination of apparently poor vision, nystagmus, eye rubbing, poor pupil light responses and a relatively normal retinal appearance will usually lead the ophthalmologist to investigate by means of the electrical tests explained in Chapter 2 (page 51). The ERG is severely affected in Leber's amaurosis and performing the test in the light and dark helps distinguish the condition from congenital stationary night blindness or achromatopsia (see previous section) which may otherwise look similar.

Medical treatment: As for all retinal dystrophies there is no treatment available at present for the basic underlying condition of the rods and cones and so medical care is limited to treating any associated refractive errors or cataract (if appropriate).

Progression: The disorder is progressive in some cases. In other cases however, an unexpected improvement of vision can take place during the first few years of life.

Educational implications: These children have at best severe visual impairment involving acuity and field and often are completely blind, and need to use braille. The fact that most of these children will never have experienced useful vision will have an effect on their concept of the world and the way they learn compared to those who have become progressively blind at an older age as, for example, in some cases of retinitis pigmentosa.

f) Retinitis Pigmentosa (RP) (Plate 31)

Definition: A group of genetic conditions initially involving progressive night blindness and peripheral visual field loss and in some cases progressing to loss of vision. The condition may be confined to the eye or part of a more widespread disorder affecting other parts of the body.

Cause: This is genetic and it can be inherited in a dominant, recessive or sex-linked way. The recessive and sex-linked types tend to come on at an earlier age and to affect vision more severely than the dominant types.

Eye structures affected: It is the rods of the retina which are primarily affected, though cones may be affected later. This accounts for the poor night vision and loss of peripheral vision as early symptoms, and the later involvement of central vision. The appearance of the retina when examined by the ophthalmologist gives a black speckled pattern, paleness of the optic disc (since the nerve fibres of the ganglion cells which make up the optic disc gradually die off as a result of the retinal damage) and narrowing of the blood vessels which supply the retina.

Apart from the primary retinal problem, cataract may develop and also the macula of the retina may become waterlogged (called macular oedema).

Effect on vision: The early problems comprise reduced vision in poor light and reduced peripheral visual field. Early visual field defects tend to be in the upper field but these gradually grow to give a ring shaped field defect (ring scotoma). Further progression in the more severe cases may lead to only a tunnel of central vision remaining (**Plate 12**). Central vision may be affected by progressive involvement of the cones in the disease or by cataract or macular oedema (see above).

Other associations: There are a number of syndromes associated with RP-like retinal dystrophies and they are outlined here:

i) Abetalipoproteinaemia

This is a rare, recessively inherited condition affecting the way fat is absorbed into the bloodstream from the diet and can also produce a disorder of balance because the balance part of the brain (the cerebellum) is affected in addition to the retinal dystrophy.

ii) Refsum's disease

This is another rare, recessively inherited condition due to a biochemical abnormality and producing an RP-like condition as well as a cerebellar disorder causing balance problems and damage to the nerves running throughout the body to and from the brain. Other features can include an absent or reduced sense of smell, deafness and heart problems. Night blindness is a common early symptom but the condition is not usually diagnosed until early adult life. Special dietary restrictions (for example, avoiding meat from grazing animals) may prevent many of the above features but the effect of diet on the progression of the retinal disease and deafness is not certain. A rare form of the disease comes on in infancy.

iii) Usher's syndrome

Again, this is usually a recessively inherited disease featuring severe hearing loss from birth as well as RP. It is the most common of the various syndromes associated with RP. Because the severe deafness can be present from birth, normal speech rarely develops. Night blindness is usually reported in late childhood or early teens and often reasonable acuity is maintained throughout the school years but may deteriorate to 6/60 or worse by middle age. It is now clear that there are different types of Usher's disease. Type 1 involves profound deafness from birth with no intelligible speech. Balance problems and learning difficulties may be additional features. Type 2 Usher's disease involves less severe hearing and retinal problems and speech may be present. It should be noted that although Usher's is the best known cause of visual and hearing impairment, a number of the syndromes outlined in this section can produce hearing loss in conjunction with retinitis pigmentosa. Congenital rubella can also cause these problems together though the retinal condition is unlikely to be progressive in rubella.

iv) Kearns–Sayre syndrome

This is a disease affecting different parts of the body in different ways. It is inherited in an unusual pattern through the mother who is usually an unaffected carrier of the disorder (maternal inheritance, see glossary). Heart rhythm problems can sometimes occur and other features can include brain, muscle and kidney disorders. The eye problems include an RP like dystrophy and progressive limitation of the movements of the eyes which is due to damage of the fibres of the six muscles which move each eye.

v) Cockayne's syndrome

Again rare and recessively inherited, this condition involves growth retardation, deafness, a physical appearance of being older than the child's actual age, learning difficulties and RP. In most cases visual and general development is normal during the first year of life, following which there is slow physical and intellectual deterioration with a life expectancy of between ten and thirty years. Additional abnormalities of the eye can include corneal opacity, cataract and nystagmus.

vi) Joubert's syndrome

This recessively inherited condition involves:
a) underdevelopment of a part of the brain used for control of movement called the cerebellum;
b) a retinal dystrophy;

c) breathing difficulties as a baby;

d) disturbance of eye movement.

The retinal dystrophy is similar to Leber's amaurosis in infancy but the visual outlook is better with the acuity sometimes reaching 6/18. The cerebellar abnormality will affect the child's ability to learn to perform tasks involving movement and control of the muscles.

vii) Mucopolysaccharidoses

An RP like dystrophy can develop in most of these conditions (described in the section on 'biochemical disorders'.)

How it is detected: The condition may be diagnosed at various ages depending on its severity. The child will usually describe difficulty seeing in the dark. Older patients may present when they notice their field of vision becoming increasingly constricted (by which time they often have severe visual field loss). Examination reveals the signs mentioned above and the diagnosis is confirmed by performing an ERG (see Chapter 2, page 51) which has a characteristically reduced result especially in the dark.

Medical treatment: There is no specific treatment for retinitis pigmentosa except in the case of Refsum's disease and abetalipoproteinaemia. Medical care may initially be limited to full and sympathetic explanations together with genetic counselling. Macular oedema is sometimes treated with medication such as steroids and cataract surgery is sometimes required, though not usually in childhood.

Progression: This varies according to the type of the disease. Sex-linked cases of retinitis pigmentosa are night blind in early childhood, and tend to show extensive field loss by the early teens and central visual loss in the twenties. By the fourth decade most patients have vision reduced to less than the ability to count fingers. The recessive form is extremely variable but is usually early in onset and severe. The outlook is much better in the dominant form in which night blindness and field loss may develop in childhood, but in the long term most patients retain reasonable visual acuity until the age of forty or fifty or even throughout life.

Educational implications: It must be remembered that most children with RP will have quite restricted visual fields despite reasonable acuity, and that this has implications for the way in which the learning environment in the classroom should be set up, and for the child's ability to navigate through the environment as he or she moves around. Obviously, lighting levels must be adequate since vision is poor in dim lighting. Ironically many RP children have poor vision in bright sunlight and have problems in adapting from bright to dim illumination. Tinted lenses can be helpful in this respect, especially in summer. The most severe cases will have reduction in acuity even at school age and Low Vision Aids (LVAs) may be required.

g) Macular dystrophies

Definition: These are a group of inherited disorders where the central part of the retina responsible for central vision and visual acuity (the macula) is predominantly affected.

Cause: The cause is genetic, and both dominant and recessive forms of inheritance are seen.

Eye structures affected: By definition it is the macula which is primarily affected.

Effect on vision: The typical picture is of gradual onset loss of visual acuity in both eyes during the first two decades of life. The degree of acuity loss is variable. In one type of macular dystrophy, Best's disease (which is dominantly inherited), most people keep reasonable reading vision until adult life. Another type, called Stargardt's disease (usually recessively inherited) involves gradual deterioration of acuity to the 6/60 or 'count fingers' level in most patients though acuity may only be mildly reduced at the outset (see page 39). Colour vision is usually normal early in the disease but becomes abnormal as the macular damage progresses. Peripheral visual fields are usually well maintained in these conditions since the peripheral retina is unaffected. It is appropriate to mention another condition called 'juvenile retinoschisis' in this section. It is not strictly a macular dystrophy but the main effect on vision is from damage to the macula which involves splitting of the layers of the retina in the macular region (hence the name schisis). It is inherited in an X-linked pattern and only boys are affected. It is often picked up between the ages of 5 and 10 causing reading difficulties or failure of the school eye test. Visual acuities are usually in the range of 6/12 to 6/36 at presentation and the outlook for vision is quite reasonable, progression being slow.

Other associations: These disorders are not associated with abnormalities in other parts of the body.

How it is detected: There is often a characteristic appearance of the macula when it is viewed with an ophthalmoscope. For instance, there is a yellow discoloration of the macula in Best's disease which is said to resemble egg yolk (hence its alternative name of vitelliform dystrophy from the Latin for 'yolk'). Electrical tests of the retina as outlined in Chapter 2 (page 51) can be helpful in making the diagnosis.

Medical treatment: No specific medical treatments are yet available. Genetic counselling is important for the families of these children as in all cases of inherited disorders of vision.

Progression: Slow deterioration through life is the general rule, though the speed and degree of this deterioration is variable.

Educational implications: Those children with more severe macular damage may benefit from the use of Low Vision Aids (LVAs). As the condition tends to progress gradually during school-age years, during which time educational material becomes progressively more detailed, a time can be reached when the child starts to experience visual difficulties. It is important to watch out for this problem. Initially, it remains possible to read but it takes longer. This can be associated with frustration, falling behind, and on occasion, challenging behaviour. Enlargement of educational material, where appropriate, and other strategies such as LVAs will help to address these problems.

h) Norrie's disease and incontinentia pigmenti

Definition: Both are rare genetic disorders involving incorrect development of the vitreous jelly and retina.

Cause: Both are inherited in an X-linked pattern, but Norrie's disease only affects boys and incontinentia pigmenti only affects girls (since it is fatal in boys).

Eye structures affected: The eyes are affected in all cases of Norrie's disease, but only in about 35% of cases of incontinentia pigmenti. Because of the abnormalities of the vitreous and retina the pupil may appear white.

Effect on vision: Children with Norrie's disease are blind from birth or early infancy, whereas children with incontinentia pigmenti may retain varying degrees of vision.

Other associations:
Norrie's disease: About a quarter of children have learning difficulties and about a third have hearing problems which may develop at any time from infancy to adult life.

Incontinentia pigmenti: The skin (with unusual linear patterns of discolouration), bones, teeth, and brain can all be affected.

How it is detected: The unusual combinations of symptoms usually lead to diagnosis in early infancy.

Medical treatment: Children with incontinentia pigmenti should be seen at regular intervals by ophthalmologists since it is possible that early treatment of the retina with a laser or a freezing probe may prevent progression of the disease.

Progression: Although some progression may be seen in incontinentia pigmenti, which may be preventable by treatment, progression is not a major feature of either of these conditions.

Educational implications: Children with Norrie's disease may need to have access to learning braille or a tactile alphabet such as Moon where appropriate, although additional learning and hearing difficulties may present further challenges in their education.

i) Batten's disease

Definition: A progressive condition involving blindness, epileptic seizures and mental deterioration.

Cause: This is a genetic disorder inherited in a recessive pattern. If certain blood cells are examined under a microscope they are seen to contain packets of an abnormal substance. This is because the abnormal gene which causes the disease affects the ability of the body to eliminate a particular fat-like substance. Brain and retinal cells therefore become loaded with this substance causing damage. The exact biochemical nature of this substance has yet to be identified.

Eye structures affected: Initially the macula and soon the whole retina is affected. Ophthalmoscopic examination reveals a characteristic 'bull's eye' appearance of the macula early on in the disease, and later on generalised pigment speckling, pallor of the optic disc and thinning of the retinal arteries (as in retinitis pigmentosa) may all be seen. Although it is the retina which is primarily affected and responsible for the poor vision, keratoconus and cataract may be additional features.

Effect on vision: Children usually present with failing vision between the ages of 4 and 10. One characteristic finding at presentation is eccentric viewing, with the child tending to look above the target, which may be due to relative preservation of the upper retina (if the child fixes above the target, light rays from the target will strike the upper retina). Children usually become functionally blind within three years of diagnosis.

Other associations: Mental deterioration and behavioural disturbance occur early, often predating visual deterioration. The epileptic seizures usually begin between the ages of 7 and 16.

How it is detected: The combination of the bull's eye macular appearance, the fits and the mental deterioration are suggestive of the diagnosis. Electrical tests of vision show characteristic abnormalities and a brain scan shows some thinning of the brain. The microscopic appearance of certain blood cells is also abnormal as described above.

Medical treatment: Anti-convulsant medication is usually successful in controlling the seizures. No other specific treatments are presently available.

Progression: The disease follows a slow downward path with dementia occurring in the teens and death sometimes well into the second or third decade.

Educational implications: Blindness is invariable and therefore access to braille may be appropriate. Additional challenges are presented by the progressive learning difficulties and the seizures.

Chronic anti-convulsant medication will be required and side effects such as occasional drowsiness may result. The adverse prognosis will obviously have an effect on the family and their attitude to the child's education.

NB Other rare biochemical storage diseases with similar features to Batten's disease (visual impairment, learning difficulty and seizures) include Tay-Sachs disease and Nieman-Pick disease. A slightly different but related group of biochemical storage disorders (the leucodystrophies) primarily affect a different type of brain cell. In these conditions, difficulties in movement and clumsiness may be more of a feature than seizures or learning difficulties. Optic atrophy and cortical visual impairment can occur in the leucodystrophies.

THE SEEING NERVES

a) Optic nerve hypoplasia
b) Optic atrophy

a) Optic nerve hypoplasia

Definition: Congenital underdevelopment of one or both optic nerves, so that the optic nerve head appears small on ophthalmoscopic examination.

Cause: In the majority of cases, no cause is identified. Maternal diabetes or alcohol abuse, generalised brain damage, and genetic causes can contribute to the development of this disorder. The common link is that something disturbs the development of the optic nerve at an early stage of the embryo in the uterus.

Eye structures affected: Primarily it is the optic nerve. Secondary features may include nystagmus and squint.

Effect on vision: This is variable and depends on the severity of the condition and whether one or both eyes are involved. Severe hypoplasia causes blindness and this condition is now a significant and possibly increasing cause of childhood visual impairment. Some children with lesser degrees of hypoplasia may have reasonable acuities but visual field defects, while others may appear to have normal vision.

Other associations: This condition may sometimes be associated with more generalised brain damage or underdevelopment. One specific association with bilateral optic nerve hypoplasia is called septo-optic dysplasia and can involve underdevelopment of some of the middle parts of the brain including the central connections between the left and right sides of the brain and hormonal centres responsible for control of growth and sexual development.

How it is detected: It is detected by ophthalmoscopic examination which reveals that the optic nerve head is smaller than usual. This is sometimes a difficult sign to pick up and the diagnosis is sometimes missed initially.

Medical treatment: Associated abnormalities such as a lack of hormones in septo-optic dysplasia may require specific medical treatment.

Progression: This is a non-progressive condition.

Educational implications: These depend on the severity of the visual impairment and on the presence of any associated developmental delay. Patients with both nerves affected may have some degree of associated brain damage, particularly the central connections between the left and right brain, which may produce subtle or marked learning difficulties. This condition may also be associated with more profound disorders of brain growth and development which may predispose to a wide range of special needs.

b) Optic atrophy

Definition: A group of diseases involving damage to the nerve fibres of the optic nerve which normally transmit signals from the retina to the visual brain.

Cause: The cause is usually genetic and the type of inheritance varies. Dominant inheritance is the most common and tends to be associated with milder visual impairment than the rarer recessively inherited optic atrophy. Leber's optic neuropathy (completely different from Leber's amaurosis) has an unusual genetic inheritance whereby it is only transmitted through the mother and more commonly affects males, usually as teenagers or young adults. Other causes for such damage to the optic nerves include poisonous side effects of certain rarely used drugs or exposure to heavy metals such as lead. Pressure from a tumour or invasion from a cancer such as leukaemia can damage the optic nerves as can a severe head injury, particularly if the skull is fractured near the small openings at the back of the orbits through which the nerves pass towards the brain.

Eye structures affected: The optic nerves are the only structures usually affected.

Effect on vision: Children with dominant optic atrophy usually present before the age of ten often at the school eye test with symmetrical mildly reduced acuities in the range of 6/9 to 6/24. Visual field defects may affect both fixation and enlargement of the normal blind spot (centrocaecal scotoma). Blue-yellow colour vision defects may also be present. Leber's optic neuropathy tends not to present until the late teens with fairly sudden and profound loss of central vision in one eye, followed shortly thereafter by the other eye. Limited but useful recovery may occur over the following two years. DIDMOAD syndrome (see below) is a rare condition which produces severe but not total loss of central vision and colour blindness. One specific type of visual field loss occurs when the optic atrophy is caused by a tumour pressing at the crossover of the optic nerves (optic chiasm). It is the nerve fibres from the nasal side of each retina which cross over and it is these fibres which are damaged. The nasal part of the retina corresponds to the outer (temporal) part of visual space and hence it is the outer part of the visual field which is damaged in both eyes (called a bitemporal hemianopia), leaving only a narrow strip of vision in the centre. A child with such a bitemporal hemianopia may complain that objects disappear because there is a segment of blindness arising from overlap of the temporal field defects beyond the object of interest, and may show behaviour consistent with this observation.

Other associations: Wasting of the optic nerves (optic atrophy) may occur in association with a number of other illnesses. DIDMOAD syndrome (Diabetes Insipidus, Diabetes Mellitus, Optic Atrophy, Deafness) consists of two types of diabetes as well as both visual and hearing impairment. There is a group of inherited diseases involving the brain and spinal cord and which cause learning difficulties, and difficulties in controlling posture and movement, which may also be accompanied by optic atrophy. Such diseases include Behr's disease, Friedreich's ataxia and others.

How it is detected: Instead of having a normal healthy pink appearance, the optic nerve heads appear pale and white when examined with the ophthalmoscope. Electrical tests may also help make the diagnosis.

Medical treatment: Any cause for the wasting of the nerves such as a tumour, malnutrition or poisoning must be removed if possible. Any additional abnormalities such as diabetes must also be appropriately treated. There is no successful medical treatment for the optic atrophy itself.

Progression: As already mentioned this is variable. Dominant optic atrophy is only slowly progressive and usually mild, whereas Leber's optic neuropathy is characterised by rapid onset severe visual loss with only limited if any recovery.

Educational implications: The type of educational material appropriate will depend on the acuity and contrast sensitivity. Teachers should also be aware of the visual field defects (peripheral vision is often reasonably good) and of the colour vision defects (more often blue-yellow). Good lighting increases reading speed in most forms of optic atrophy.

THE SEEING BRAIN

a) Cortical visual impairment
b) Hydrocephalus

a) Cortical visual impairment

Definition: Impairment of vision due to brain damage affecting the visual cortex or the pathways within the brain.

Cause: The most common cause of this condition is inadequate oxygen reaching the brain around the time of birth. Premature babies are particularly vulnerable to this type of injury (since the blood vessels supplying parts of the brain are fragile). Since more infants are now surviving due to improved medical care, the incidence of cortical blindness is increasing, and probably now represents the most common cause of visual impairment in children in developed countries.

Other causes of damage to the visual brain include accidental or non-accidental head injury, infection such as meningitis and, as described in the following section, hydrocephalus.

Eye structures affected: In general the eyes themselves are unaffected, though there may be disordered control of eye movement (with difficulty in tracking moving objects), or squint present.

Effect on vision: This can range from the subtle defects of complex visual processing to complete absence of functional vision, depending upon the site and extent of the brain damage. One-sided field defects (hemianopias) may occur if the damage is asymmetrical. Damage to the left visual brain results in absent or disordered vision on the right side and vice versa. If the damage has been caused by an interruption of the blood supply to the brain there may be sparing of central vision despite severe damage to the peripheral fields on one side or the other. This phenomenon is called macular sparing and is thought to arise because the part of the visual cortex corresponding to the maculae (and hence central vision), which is situated right at the back of the brain, has a spare blood supply to keep it going if the main supply is damaged.

Cortically blind children may navigate comfortably round objects of furniture and show awareness of moving objects surprisingly accurately even though they appear blind when their vision is tested by normal methods. This form of subconscious vision is called blindsight and is thought to arise from the alternative visual pathway which never reaches the visual cortex and hence never reaches consciousness. This pathway is faster than the cortical pathway and is specially adapted for navigational tasks involving perception of movement (stationary furniture is moving visually when a child moves past it). This form of vision is present in human beings and most other species. It is more highly developed in animals such as birds which have to fly through trees at high speeds without crashing and where fast visual reflexes are essential. This type of vision may not be apparent at birth or even during the first two or three years of life. However, gradual development of navigational vision may take place during the ensuing years. Different aspects of visual processing such as the recognition of motion and recognition of geometric shapes or faces, occur at different sites in the visual cortex, some predominantly in one side of the brain (eg face recognition on the right side, and reading vision on the left) and other aspects of vision on both sides (eg colour and movement perception). The specific weakness of one such aspect of visual processing is called a visual agnosia. For example, inability to recognise faces is called prosopagnosia. Many of these agnosias are still being discovered and defined but they clearly have a profound effect on the way a child handles visual educational material. **Figure 1.6** (page 25) illustrates some of the agnosias which are known to be associated with damage to particular areas of the brain. This information has come from carefully assessing patients' visual capabilities, identifying a particular weakness and looking at brain scans to locate the site of the brain damage. For example it has been found that patients with prosopagnosia commonly have damage to one particular site in the right side of the brain near the back, and so we conclude that the processing of face recognition occurs in this site in the brain.

Other associations: Learning difficulties, posture and movement difficulties (cerebral palsy), seizures and hydrocephalus may all accompany the visual problems in these cases.

How it is detected: The child has visual problems but examination of the eyes themselves reveals no abnormality. Scans of the brain are good at showing up areas of damage and can enable doctors to localise the areas of damage which may give clues as to what type of visual disorders to look for. Children with cognitive visual impairment tend not to be aware that they have a visual problem. Damage to a part of the brain for a specific visual function is associated with damage to the part of the brain responsible for knowing and understanding that function, so that the affected person is not aware of her deficiency. The diagnosis is therefore made by watching the child's visual behaviour and identifying specific inconsistencies of this behaviour.

Medical treatment: No specific treatment is available once the damage is sustained and medical care of vulnerable neonates and infants is directed at trying to reduce the risk and severity of the brain damage occurring in the first place.

Progression: Episodes of cortical visual impairment may be temporary, though complete restoration of vision is unusual. Gradual improvement of visual function may be slow, taking months to years. One study found that cortically blind children often had no light perception initially and with time gained colour vision, form perception and finally, improved visual acuity. Some degree of visual agnosia often remains, however.

Educational implications: These children often have a short visual attention span and their visual skills often seem to vary from minute to minute which can cause confusion to carers - tiredness and overly complex visual information can impede visual perception. Colour vision sometimes appears to be better preserved than vision for shapes and form, and children may be attracted to red and yellow objects in particular. This may be because colour vision is processed on both sides of the brain and so even if damage is sustained to one side, there may be some remaining *'spare'* brain on the other side for processing colour. It will therefore be helpful to represent shapes and letters being taught to the child in colour against a highly contrasting and uncluttered background. Children with hemianopias may turn their head to the side when reaching for objects in order to use the good side of their visual field.

Cortically visually impaired children may find it easier to view educational material at a closer range than would be expected. In addition to magnifying the target (the closer you move your eyes to an object, the bigger it becomes) this also reduces the amount of visual information to be processed (the closer you move your eyes to an object, the fewer additional objects there are round the edges of the picture). The reduction in visual performance due to too much visual information is called 'crowding' and teachers should be aware of the limits of the amount of visual information that can be taken in by the child at one time.

A typical example in a younger child is the inability to find a toy on a patterned carpet but the ability to find it on a plain one. A cortically visually impaired child may need to be presented with visual targets one at a time whereas children with other forms of visual impairment may be able to perceive a number of targets simultaneously. Another strategy which may help the child overcome this crowding phenomenon is to trace or follow objects with a finger.

An analogy which illustrates the impairment of processing would be to consider the effect on supermarket queues if, instead of having ten checkout counters working simultaneously, nine of them went out of order and all the customers had to pass through the same counter, one after the other. This lack of ability to parallel process visual information has a profound effect on the way in which visual tasks and processes are learned.

If, for instance, a simple task such as dressing a doll is considered, a child will typically learn to do this by seeing the doll and the dress and imagining simultaneously in his or her mind's eye the doll with the dress on, so that he or she knows what the next stage of the task involves. A cortically visually impaired child may not be able simultaneously to perceive the doll, the dress and the imagined dressed doll and hence will need to be taught to perform the task in a stepwise manner by imitation, with repetition and gradually more of the task being performed by the child him/herself. This will be quite time consuming, especially when more visually complex educational tasks are taught and learned. It is important not to expect the same speed of performance from children with cortical visual impairment as those children in the same class with visual impairment resulting from eye disease.

Some children like to gaze at bright lights, even to the point of gazing into the sun which should be discouraged by the carer because of the risk of burns to the retina. Paradoxically, other children with this condition are distressed by bright light (photophobia).

Some educational strategies which have been found to be helpful in dealing with some of the specific visual problems experienced by many of these children are outlined here:

i) Problems with recognition

In order to recognise somebody or something we have to keep a store of the pictures we have seen in the past. Recognition is the result of an image which we see matching an image in our memory. If there is a match, the image is recognised. If there is no match, the image is explored (using all the senses in harmony) ready for future recognition. This is a complex task and different parts of the brain are responsible for different recognition processes. As has already been mentioned, the right part of the brain at the back (also responsible for seeing on the left hand side) is responsible for recognising faces, and damage to this area can cause difficulty in recognising faces (prosopagnosia). This is usually compensated for by voice recognition, but training in memorising certain dressing features or other characteristics can prove helpful.

The back of the brain on the left (also responsible for seeing on the right hand side) has a major role for the recognition of shape and form. Children with difficulty in this territory often have difficulties with jigsaws, and in understanding and interpreting three-dimensional images.

Difficulty in reading (dyslexia) or inability to read (alexia) in children with cortical visual impairment may occur in those who have difficulty seeing on the right side. For these children the principal problem is one of converting the written word into a real (or imagined) sound otherwise known as a phoneme. The basis of the strategies required to overcome this problem is to use visual pattern recognition in the same way as Chinese is taught. For example, the child can be encouraged to build up a dictionary of his or her own words upon which they have imposed their own pictures. Rapid *'look and see'* reading in which the meaning is extracted but without reading out loud is a useful strategy to attempt in this unusual situation.

ii) <u>Problems with orientation</u>
This is more common in individuals with damage to the back of the brain on the right. In order to find your way around you need to have a route map in your memory which can be matched to the world outside. Some children with cortical visual impairment have great difficulty in finding their way around, both within buildings and outside. They also have difficulty in remembering where they have put things. A wide range of strategies can be used to get round these difficulties. In the home, colour coding for different doors in the house can be used and can be gradually faded out in order to use a colour based memory system. Outside, by constantly talking about where things are as you move past them, a language based memory can be developed. On a smaller scale, problems with losing things are best circumvented by making sure that *'everything has its place'*.

iii) <u>Difficulty in seeing parts of an image against a complex background</u>
This seems to be most common in children with cerebral palsy and impairment of movement of all four limbs. Such children

appear to see a single picture fairly easily against a plain background or can find a toy on a plain carpet, but are unable to extract any meaning from the same picture set against a complex background or to find a toy on a patterned carpet. In education, the term *'figure ground'* has been used to apply to this problem.

From an educational point of view it is logical to provide small amounts of information sequentially against a plain background. Some children can be helped by masking off other words in the text. Reading, of course can be difficult and is very slow. When the purpose of reading is to learn to read, the amount of text is reduced to the amount that the child can cope with. When the purpose of reading is however to access information, use of the spoken word is more efficient.

iv) <u>Impaired depth perception</u>
As we look at the world around us we create an immediate mental pictorial image of what we see which, of course, we take for granted. This is, however, a very complicated computing task and it is not surprising that difficulties can arise due to the incomplete formation of such 3-dimensional mental images. A particular problem which such children experience is one of going down stairs or steps. On occasion, they find it very difficult to know whether a line on the floor represents a step or not. They also may have a problem in mentally constructing a three-dimensional tactile map of the world. A mobility training programme needs to take these problems, when they are present, into account.

v) <u>Impaired perception of movement</u>
This is usually seen in children with damage to the back of the brain on both sides. Children with this problem appear to have difficulty in seeing and interpreting fast movement, whether it be movement of objects past them, or their own movement through the visual world. Such children may prefer cartoon images which do not move much, such as Spot the Dog, or Thomas the Tank Engine.

It is important for teachers of visually impaired children to recognise that no two children with the same diagnostic label will experience exactly the same type of impairment of vision. This is particularly true of cortical visual impairment because of the complexity of processing which takes place in the visual brain. One child with cortical visual impairment may only see stationary objects, another may see only moving objects. Such children need to be assessed as individuals and to have their educational material presented to them in a way that matches their particular visual abilities. It is also important to recognise that the reason so much brain tissue (40%) is devoted to visual function is that our understanding, interpretation and movement through the visual world is a very complex process. A child who has sustained damage to this part of the brain at or around birth is inevitably unaware that there are any visual problems and it is only by careful observation of behaviour that it is possible to recognise that such problems exist. Moreover, because a child's brain is developing and growing, a child may well learn a range of subconscious strategies in order to either circumvent or overcome the problems. With assistance and training the child may well be able to deal with some of his or her visual problems to such an extent that they are no longer manifest a few years later.

b) Hydrocephalus

Definition: The brain contains cavities (called ventricles) into which clear fluid is pumped from the blood. The fluid passes through the cavities and then out to surround the brain like a waterbath and then is absorbed back into the bloodstream. If the fluid is not drained adequately, the pressure in the ventricles builds up (similar to inadequate drainage of aqueous fluid in the eye leading to a build up of intraocular pressure in glaucoma), the brain tissue is compressed and the size of the cavities increases. This is called 'hydrocephalus' which literally means 'water on the brain'.

Cause: A number of different problems can cause inadequate drainage of brain fluid back into the blood. The child may be born with a malformation of the brain or spinal cord such as spina bifida which causes a block to the normal passage of the brain fluid. Other causes may be acquired in infancy or childhood such as meningitis (which may leave scarring in the brain), bleeding into the brain (infants born prematurely are particularly prone to this problem) or tumours in the brain which may compress the outflow channels.

Eye structures affected: The optic nerves may show wasting or atrophy (see optic atrophy, page 105).

Effect on vision: Optic atrophy and cortical visual impairment are both common, and the effects on vision are as explained in the sections devoted to these topics. The visual parts of the brain or visual cortex may be damaged by direct pressure or by interruption to the blood supply, and in some cases by the surgery which involves insertion of a plastic bypass tube into the ventricles (possibly through areas near the visual cortex) to let the water drain out and which may be necessary to save the child's life. Control of eye position and movement is often affected in hydrocephalus. The child may be unable to move his eyes upwards and therefore have to move his or her whole head back in order to achieve this. The nerves to the muscles which move the eyes out to the side are also vulnerable to raised pressure in the brain and if they are damaged the eye may be temporarily or permanently turned in. In this instance, an older child may experience double vision, especially if both eyes see well.

Other associations: In infants the skull bones are relatively elastic and the head may be enlarged (analagous to enlargement of the eye in infantile glaucoma). In older children that elasticity is not there to accommodate the increased pressure and hence features such as headache, drowsiness, nausea and vomiting may occur in addition to any of the visual features mentioned.

How it is detected: The features already mentioned lead to suspicion of hydrocephalus and the diagnosis is confirmed with a brain scan, which clearly shows the enlarged ventricles in the brain.

Medical treatment: Surgeons can perform operations to bypass the blockage to the absorption of the brain fluid. This involves inserting a tube (called a shunt) with one end in a brain ventricle and the other end draining either directly into the heart or into the abdominal cavity from where the fluid then drains naturally back into the bloodstream. These shunts are life saving but are prone to complications such as infection or blockage. All carers and professionals involved with the child should be aware of the signs that a shunt may not be functioning properly since urgent surgical correction is often required. The signs which are indicative of raised pressure include headache, drowsiness, nausea, vomiting, visual or behavioural disturbances, or new abnormalities of eye position or movement. The shunt also has to be inserted through brain tissue which in itself may cause visual field defects or deficits of specific visual function localised to the area of cortex through which the shunt was inserted.

If eye movement or position is a problem then prisms stuck onto the surface of spectacle lenses (or incorporated into them) or even simple occlusion of one eye may alleviate double vision. Squint surgery is sometimes helpful in correcting abnormal eye position. This simply involves repositioning some of the muscles which move the eyes.

Progression: Progression of this condition can usually be avoided by appropriate surgery and careful follow up for any signs of shunt dysfunction.

Educational implications: Cortical visual impairment and optic atrophy are common, and the reader is referred to the educational implications outlined in these sections. The teacher must be aware of the signs of shunt dysfunction as explained above. Repeated hospital visits and or admissions are likely to be necessary which may potentially interfere with schooling.

CHAPTER 4

EDUCATING VISUALLY IMPAIRED CHILDREN

Children's visual problems vary from relatively minor to profound in nature. The principle challenges which teachers encounter are with those whose vision is more profoundly impaired. This chapter is primarily written with this group of children in mind. Much of what follows will be relevant to children who use braille as their main means of reading but this chapter does not attempt to cover the teaching of braille or the use of braille-related technology. The bibliography lists some books in which these topics are covered.

Before a teacher, parent or carer begins to think about the educational implications of a child's visual impairment, they must remind themselves of one important fact: any labels accompanying a child, whether it be the medical term for the visual impairment, or a clinical assessment of the child's vision, should be taken into account but not considered as prescriptive. Two children may well have the same medical condition and even the same visual acuity and yet require remarkably different support within a school.

Why is that? Many factors contribute to a child's ability to see; only one of those factors is the physical condition of the eye, or the intact pathways between the eye and the brain which enables sensory information to be interpreted. Any problem in these areas results in the visual impairment. However, the other factors which affect a child's functional vision, that is, the ability to use eyesight in everyday situations, include his or her:

- Motivation for learning
- Access to an environment which encourages use of functional vision
- Access to materials and technology which aid functional vision
- Training in the use of functional vision

Clearly, a child's medical condition is important and the term will provide useful information to the carer. For example, the implications of albinism are likely to include ensuring the child is protected from bright lighting, but the term albinism does not mean that every child with albinism will require exactly the same measure of protection. Each child's needs must be assessed individually.

If you are a fully-sighted person you will know that even your ability to see can be affected by environmental factors or personal circumstances. So, if you are very tired, perhaps ill, you will find it hard to read, to take in information and process it. Similarly, if the print of a book is too small, or you are reading in poor lighting conditions, you will find it harder both to discriminate the letters and concentrate, and so your speed of reading will decrease. Furthermore, if you are struggling to see, then your motivation to concentrate and learn will also be adversely affected. If, for example, you are in a large meeting, unable to see the facial features of the speaker clearly, then it is often harder to maintain an interest in what is being said. As your visual attention decreases, so often does your motivation to listen. Visually impaired children face these situations all the time, and yet they are not an inevitable consequence of visual impairment. Children can be trained to use their functional vision to maximum effect; their motivation can be encouraged by following simple, often common-sense principles when providing them with educational materials, planning their environment and allowing them the freedom to explore, experience and memorise this environment. Thus, the adults involved with a visually impaired child should be knowledgeable about both the visual impairment of the child and the other factors which affect his functional vision. It is these factors which are considered in this chapter.

MOTIVATION FOR LEARNING

The motivation to use the vision that is present is, in the final analysis, the responsibility of the child, but the importance of early intervention in a visually impaired child's development cannot be over-emphasised. A visually impaired baby or young child might not have the stimulus of sight to encourage him to develop all or any of the following normal steps that typically characterise development:

i)   focus on faces, objects
ii) follow movements
iii) realize an object is there and so reach out to grasp it
iv) see different facial expressions and gradually attach meaning to them
v)   see lips move and realize language is emerging
vi) realize that even if an object cannot be touched, it still exists and is still there
vii) copy movements

The importance of sensory stimulation at a young age for the development of the brain is well-known. As the visually impaired child gets little incidental motivation to use his vision, it is understandable that there may be a tendency for that child to withdraw into passivity or self-stimulation within his own body eg eye-poking, hand-flapping etc. Fully sighted babies or young children not only have a constant input of information through sight; his early communication with others is generally visual, and stimulates further development. A visually impaired child will often miss the visual clues of an adult's face eg the delighted smile at something the child has done. Instead of responding by repetition of that action and further developing it, the child may appear passive and unresponsive. This can in turn discourage the adult from further interaction with the child. It need not be so, however, if the adult is aware of this and instead uses touch or noise to communicate feelings of delight and pleasure. If the adult is also aware of the developmental needs of a sighted child, eg what stimulates him to explore and learn, then it is possible to think about how to adapt those same principles for a visually impaired child by:

- bringing objects and faces nearer
- making objects brighter
- providing greater contrast, or better lighting
- attaching noises to objects
- reducing visual crowding, for example, by presenting objects one at a time, against a suitable background.

We are not talking of expensive specialised resources, but of adapting what already exists for fully-sighted children. One excellent source of ideas and explanation for stimulating vision is *'Show Me What My Friends Can See'* by Sonksen and Stiff. As the visually impaired child gets older, he will need to have objects in the environment explained and pointed out. It will depend on each individual's intellectual ability, as well as the nature of their visual impairment, as to how often explanations need to be repeated, perhaps once, perhaps several times. Thus, a child with poor distance vision may be told one day that the large red vehicle approaching is a bus; note that the child will not necessarily know this and will need it pointed out at least once (and will have to have explored a bus to know what it is). The colour, sound and shape of the object will need to be memorised and retrieved by the child to identify a bus at a later stage. Such learning will depend on the child's ability to retain such information and use it at an appropriate time.

However, early intervention to encourage such active looking is vital. Later on, the child's sense of direction will be affected, as he will not see obstacles clearly and be able to plan routes. The child's concept of the surrounding world is also affected by visual impairment; he cannot subconsciously take in visual information and begin to build up an ordered categorization of objects. For example, it will take longer for a visually impaired child to identify the common elements of a chair, (ie it has 4 legs and is for sitting in,) and then to realize that a chair can be tall, small, made of wood or plastic and yet still remain a chair. This will probably never need to be explained to a fully-sighted child. The visually impaired child needs to explore objects by touch, trying to put the different pieces together mentally; this will take far longer than the sighted child's glance and recognition of an object.

It is important that the carer makes no assumptions about a visually impaired child's previous experiences and level of understanding about any subject, but finds out first what has been understood before moving on to the next stage, and provides enough time for the child to explore and memorise his environment. As the child realizes he can make sense of what is around him, he will be motivated to explore and learn more.

CREATING AN OPTIMUM ENVIRONMENT

The school or home environment is not usually within the direct control of the visually impaired child, but it may well be possible for the carer to adapt it to provide the best conditions for him. This will involve thinking through the following issues:

- safety
- clarity and contrast
- lighting
- ease of access for mobility and independence
- the sound environment; providing good acoustic conditions.

i)   Safety
       Every child, whether sighted or not, will learn best in a safe, secure environment. The school or home environment is not always ideal, as it often has not been designed with the visually impaired child in mind. Nevertheless, adaptations can be made, and common sense applied to improve it. Make sure that there are clear pathways and routes between areas; clear pathways will include ensuring there are no projections such as shelves at eye and head level. Be organised in storing materials and resources, so that a visually impaired child can find them without having to search in unknown places. An orderly and reasonably predictable environment will greatly enhance a child's confidence and enjoyment in the learning situation. Be aware of such hazards as trailing leads, or ill-fitting carpets which might cause the child to trip. Encourage the child to explore his environment and get to learn routes between various places. If a visually impaired child is coming to a new school, it is a good idea if he can visit beforehand during the holidays with a mobility officer and become familiar with the school lay-out and learn important routes.

ii)   Clarity and contrast
       Clarity and contrast are important in relation to printed material; they are as important in the environment. Strong

colour contrast can greatly aid orientation. Doorways can be outlined in a contrasting colour to the rest of the room, as can light switches, power points etc which are normally coloured to blend in with the room. Contrasting paint along the edges of stairs is an effective means of aiding mobility and making the environment safer; white or yellow is commonly used. The type of paint used within a room is also important, as different colours reflect different amounts of light. For example, a glossy white will reflect about 80% of the light falling on it, whereas a matt black surface reflects almost no light. As too much light or glare can add to a child's discomfort, this is a factor which should be borne in mind, especially when re-decoration is an option. Many classes and schools have labels and notices throughout, providing necessary information for sighted and visually impaired children alike. It need not be a problem to ensure such notices are clearly printed and placed at eye level, as the Royal Institute of Architects recommend; as with many of these measures, they will help the sighted child as much as the visually impaired child.

iii)   Lighting
Each individual will have different lighting needs, and whilst it may not be possible to change the environmental light, it is possible to suit task lighting to an individual's needs. Be aware of the fact that bright lighting is not necessarily the best for a visually impaired child; this will depend on his visual condition. The CIBS' (Chartered Institute for Building Services) recommendation for the proper level of illumination for near tasks is 300 lux for young, fully sighted people. For the over 60s, 450-600 lux is thought necessary, and for visually impaired people, something over 1000 lux is probably needed. However, as each visually impaired individual will vary, each person's preference should be assessed. It can be helpful to have a light meter to measure light levels in the different areas a visually impaired child may be using or passing through at school and at home.

CONDITION	LIGHTING ENVIRONMENT
Corneal opacities eg Peter's, metabolic diseases: cataract, albinism, aniridia	Avoid focal light sources in front of child which may cause glare.
Retinitis pigmentosa	Adequate general light levels essential - children have poorer vision in dark conditions. However excessively bright light sources can temporarily damage the retina and cause glare if there is associated contact.
Cone dystrophies	Excessively bright lighting causes discomfort and poorer vision, and should be avoided.
Macular disorders	Bright focal light sources placed behind child and directed onto target may improve detailed vision.
Optic nerve disease	Increased level of background lighting may be beneficial.

Positioning of task lighting is very important. It can be difficult to find the best position; if placed to the side, the light source can cause unpleasant glare in the peripheral field vision, or the head may block the light and form shadows. However, if the lighting is placed over the text, which is often best, then heat coming from the light can cause problems too. One solution is to use a fluorescent tube. It is cheap, provides diffused light and stays cool.

iv)   Ease of access for mobility and independence ✗
Orderly and predictable layouts of classrooms and school enable a visually impaired child to learn routes that remain constant. This builds up confidence and speed in moving about the learning environment. It also means a visually impaired child will be increasingly able to fetch necessary materials and resources independently. The effect of independent mobility on a child's self-esteem can be considerable and this in turn can benefit learning.

v) Sound environment: ensuring good acoustic conditions
A visually impaired child is much more reliant on other senses for input of information than sighted children, and hearing is the most important of these. It is vital then, that the child is not distracted from listening to another person, or from his own work, by unnecessary background noises. If walls and floors can be covered with sound absorbing acoustic tiles or carpets, so much the better; these will muffle background noise and allow meaningful noise to be more audible. If this isn't possible, then try to eliminate as much background noise as possible, for example from radios. Create quiet areas for private work through the use of movable screens. If possible, allow children using technology such as a Perkins brailler a designated place to work, where they feel comfortable they are not disturbing others, and they also are not disturbed in their work.

MATERIALS WHICH AID FUNCTIONAL VISION

As in the environment, the following factors are important when preparing materials for the use of visually impaired children:

i) Size of print and font
A visually impaired child's preferred size of print is usually found using a standard reading card, such as the Maclure reading types for children (**see Figure 2.4**). This gives examples of different sizes of type in decreasing size. A child will read these and decide which size print is most comfortable (**see Figure 4.1**).

The larger the print, the fewer letters can be perceived by the eye in any one position, and so the longer it can take to read. Thus, what is comfortable for a few sentences might become an unnecessarily tedious and slow process when faced with whole textbooks and novels in that size print and it might be preferable for that child to persevere with a smaller print when needing to access a lot of information.

FIGURE 4.1

N4.5
The brother and sister walked to a farm.

N8
The brother and sister walked to a farm.

N24
The brother and sister walked to a farm.

Conversely, a child might opt for a smaller size of print that is fine for a couple of sentences, but would become fatiguing when reading for sustained periods or in lighting conditions that are less than perfect. The font chosen by a child can often clarify print. The teacher should therefore test a child's preferred font and size of print over a sustained period of reading, and in different lighting conditions, ranging from the optimum to the less than satisfactory.

FIGURE 4.2 - *Different type point sizes*

12 Point	The lazy brown fox
13 Point	The lazy brown fox
14 Point	The lazy brown fox
15 Point	The lazy brown fox
16 Point	The lazy brown fox
17 Point	The lazy brown fox

It is important to make the pupil aware of the effects of sustained reading and different lighting conditions and to enable the pupil to choose the appropriate strategy by using different size print for different purposes, and to know when and how to use Low Vision Aids (LVAs). All too often, once a preferred print size has been chosen, it is used for all materials, whereas different sizes for different uses may well be better for the child. This should not be a difficulty as it only needs a change in the font or photocopier degree of enlargement. It is worth remembering that visually impaired children will often be faced with material that is not printed in their optimum size of print and font, especially outside school, and their educational training must prepare them to cope with this.

ii)   Clarity and contrast
Clarity in the material presented to visually impaired children is essential. Illegible writing, diagrams and graphics which overlap, smudged or faded print, all hamper their ability to see, whereas material which has been clearly printed and laid out may mean a same child who is partially sighted has equal access to material as his sighted peers. There are general principles on preparing printed texts for visually impaired children which are simple to put into practice and will probably also benefit those who are fully-sighted.

- Black against white generally though not invariably gives the best contrast.
- Where possible, avoid writing in block capitals. Words are read by recognising the overall shapes, rather than by reading letter by letter. An upper and lower case mix gives the reader the benefit of visual clues and so speeds up the process of reading.
- Printed text rather than cursive handwriting is often easier for visually impaired children to read.
- Choose paper with a matt surface, as a glossy paper can give glare from reflected focal lighting. Glare can also be a problem with white boards.

- Content layout is important. Headings and paragraphs should be left justified. Leave a line space between paragraphs and between questions.
- Key in the number/letter of a question, then tab the text. This helps the reader, if moving from question paper to exercise book, to find the relevant question again quickly.
- Where brackets are used, leave a space between brackets and text, so that the visually impaired child doesn't try to read the brackets as part of the text.
- Try to keep whole questions together on one page. If the text or question refers to a diagram or table, try to have that information facing the question, so that the visually impaired children are not having to cope with turning over pages and trying to find the right place again.
- In mathematics, it is sometimes worth using a larger print size for the division sign, as pupils often misread this for a plus sign.
- Avoid unnecessary pictures and diagrams, and decorative fonts. Most readers benefit from having less, rather than more, text and graphics on a page.

Contrast is an important factor not only in printed materials but also on the screens, or visual displays of the technology used by visually impaired children. Firstly, think about the background and the text colour. Is there clear contrast or does the text merge into the background? If colour is used, is it chosen with visually impaired children in mind? Pastel shades can be very indistinct, although to the sighted person they may be aesthetically pleasing. Where contrast is adjustable such as on CCTVs and computers, allow the visually impaired child to choose their preferred setting. Many visually impaired children favour white text on a black background, as it gives a good contrast and produces less glare than a white background.

iii) <u>Best use of colour</u>

Colour confusion is a common additional impairment to many conditions which reduce vision, but is one often ignored by professionals working with visually impaired children, because it usually doesn't have educational implications (as long as the points made previously about contrast and clarity are borne in mind). However, there are simple tests such as the Ishihara colour test which indicate which colours cause particular confusion, and these colour combinations can be avoided when preparing materials. This is perhaps more important with primary school age children.

Certain conditions, such as cortical visual impairment (CVI), do not necessarily imply accompanying colour confusion, and so children with CVI are as attracted to primary colours, such as yellow and red, as their fully-sighted peers. Experimental data suggests that the use of colour helps the perception of forms by children with CVI. This has implications for teachers who work with such children; a simple method of outlining shapes and letters with colour makes it easier for the child to perceive, and hence progress in learning. The same principle applies when it is obvious that certain colour boundaries are not seen - for example a dark green frog on light green grass. In that case, a line in a bright contrasting colour to highlight appropriate boundaries may be helpful.

Specialist technology

Technological advances mean that a child with little or no useful vision can work well within a mainstream class. Equipment includes computers that translate print into braille, that can speak out the text, personal note-takers that can produce both braille and print, Closed Circuit TVs (CCTVs) that allow access to print and diagrams. Increasingly, there is a wider range of machines on offer that can perform similar functions, so it is important that advice is sought from the appropriate advisory and support services as to what particular piece of equipment would best suit each visually impaired child's needs. The requirements of professional back-up in the form of training and maintenance should also be planned and budgeted for, as they can often prove to be as expensive as the purchase of the equipment. However, many Low Vision Aids (LVAs) for visually impaired children are much simpler and therefore cheaper. Despite their relative simplicity, though, they are often not used to any effect because the carer and the child have not received even basic training in their use, perhaps because it is assumed that their function is self-explanatory. This is not the case: the following section presents the range of LVAs commonly found in schools, and describes how they should be used.

i) <u>Hand-held Low Vision Aids (LVAs)</u>
LVA is by itself a very broad term. It can apply to anything that improves a person's visual functioning, and so can include tinted lenses, extra lighting, or hand-held magnifiers. However, the following applies to hand-held optical LVAs ie those LVAs which use lenses (**see Plate 32** for different examples).

The purpose of most optical LVAs is simply to magnify the detail of an object to a size which the visually impaired child finds easier to see. There are various ways of achieving this magnification:

- increase the size of the object eg enlarge print, diagrams etc
- decrease the working distance. Children have greater accommodation than adults and can move objects closer to the eye
- use an LVA

To use an LVA effectively, and to avoid frustration, it is important for the child to learn how to use it properly. The LVAs used for near vision must be held at the correct distance. The amount of magnification and the size of the field of view decrease as the distance from the magnifier to the eye increases. Therefore, as a general rule, magnifiers should be used close to the eye (**see Plate 33**). To keep the LVA at the correct distance from the text, it is helpful to put the little finger down on the text to act as a support and maintain the distance. In order to make reading comfortable, it is important that the printed material is brought up to the child's face, rather than the child having to bend over to the table. Wooden stands or angle-poise book-holders can be used for this.

Using the LVA
The child will need to practise:
- finding the start of the line
- tracking along and back a line
- dropping down lines
- scanning text
- developing speed and fluency in using the LVA
- cleaning and maintaining the LVA

When using the far distance LVAs such as telescopes, the child will need to practise the above skills as well as the following:
- locating objects
- focusing
- scanning along a blackboard

Choosing the right magnification
The number on the box accompanying the LVA indicates the focusing power of the LVA (measured in units called dioptres, abbreviated to 'D') and this can be used to calculate the amount of magnification. Thus, if the focusing power is + 16 D, the magnifying power of the LVA can be worked out by the following formula:

magnification = focusing power/4

In the above example, the magnification would be 16/4 = 4 and would thus magnify the image by a factor of 4, or x4.

However, this is a simplified formula, and does not take into account the working distance at which the LVA is being used. It is important to remember that generally, as the working distance increases, so the magnification of the LVA decreases. Hence the magnification calculated should be taken only as a rough guide.

Field of view must also be considered. For a near vision magnifier, field of view can be defined as the number of letters that can be seen at one time through the magnifier. It is important to note that the narrower the field, the harder it is to read whole words, and thus read quickly, and to find one's way around a page. This effect is illustrated with a map in **Plate 34**. This should therefore be borne in mind when deciding the strength of magnification, so that the size of letter is balanced by the field of view.

The width of field of view can be affected by:
- The working distance between the LVA and the eyes. The shorter the working distance, the greater the field of view.
- The diameter of the magnifying lens. The larger it is, the greater the field of view.
- The magnification rating of the lens. The lower the rating, the greater the field of view.

Types of hand-held LVAs and their use

a)   SIMPLE MAGNIFIERS:

- *Hand-held:* the user has to find the correct distance from the page, and has to maintain the position. The eyes must be close to the lens, so a work-stand that brings the material up to the face may help with posture.
  Limitation: it is not possible to write easily underneath this LVA.

- *Stand magnifier* **(Plate 35)**: the stand has the advantage of maintaining the correct distance from the page.
  Limitation: the user can't easily write underneath it, and if it doesn't have its own illumination, then shadows are cast.

- *Flat field:* these have excellent light gathering properties, and less distortion than the above LVAs. *Limitation:* they are limited to x2 magnification and do not allow writing underneath; they can only be used for reading.

- *Bar magnifiers:* these have excellent light gathering properties.
  Limitation: they only magnify the height of letters, not the width, and are generally limited to x2 magnification. They are only useful for reading.

- *Spectacle mounted magnifiers* **(Plate 36)**: the great advantage of these is that they keep both hands free, and allow the user to both read and write. They also provide maximum field of view for near vision. *Limitation:* they have a short working distance, so it is important that task lighting illuminates the work.

  Bi-focals are useful when needing to focus on close work eg reading and writing and distance work, eg looking up at a blackboard to copy. They are not usually recommended for use in walking around, although in practice, many children seem to manage.

b)   TELESCOPIC SYSTEMS **(Plate 37)**:

Telescopes for both near and distance vision are available; some models have focusing power for both near and distance work.

Example of magnification rating: 6 x 16

The first figure indicates the magnification rating, and the second indicates the diameter of the front lens in millimetres. This affects the light-gathering properties of the lens; the wider, the better. As magnification increases, the field of view decreases. Telescopes are therefore sometimes prescribed with less than maximum magnification in order to allow the user the benefit of a greater field of view.

Optical LVAs can be the correct magnification for the child, and the child may be well-trained in their correct use, but their effectiveness will be nullified if lighting is poor. Optical LVAs tend to require task lighting.

All adults concerned with the child should be aware how the LVAs should be used. Teachers, parents and carers can encourage the child to use the LVA correctly, ie at the right distance, with the appropriate lighting and posture. It is worth assessing children's use of LVAs regularly to ensure that they are still benefiting from them. If there are problems, these should be addressed before the child becomes discouraged and reluctant to use any type of LVA.

c) CLOSED CIRCUIT TVS OR CCTVs **(Plate 38)**

CCTVs can be used for reading print and diagrams. They usually consist of a camera, a platform on which the material to be read rests, and a screen. Some CCTV systems are also able to focus on material at a distance, for example on the blackboard or whiteboard. The advantages of a CCTV over a hand-held LVA are many:

- The degree of magnification is greater.
- The user can control the degree of magnification. This is more flexible when faced with textbooks with varying print sizes.
- The user can adjust the contrast and brightness.
- The picture can be reversed, to provide, for example, white against a black background.
- Other facilities such as line markers or split-screen (blacking out the text except for the line to be read) help the user track along a line and read more quickly.

CCTVs are expensive and cannot always be transported to every room by trolley. However, many schools make arrangements for a CCTV to be available for as many lessons as possible. They can be particularly useful for science and geography where sighted pupils can also benefit from the magnification of diagrams. In addition CCTVs are often made available in a resource area. A hand-held CCTV could also be an option where portability is a factor, although these can be more difficult to use and may be more appropriate for secondary school pupils.

The training skills outlined for using hand-held LVAs will apply to using CCTVs.

Techniques relevant to CCTVs will also need to be mastered by a child:

- Camera controls: print size
  focusing
  zooming
- Screen: contrast
  brightness
  positive/negative image
  line marker, split screen
  facility using the platform to move work

The child will gain confidence in using a CCTV through careful explanation of all the controls and practise in using them. Teachers may find it helpful to have a collection of different types of print eg text in columns, drawings, comics, photos, graphs, maps and a selection of different print sizes and styles so that the child can get used to changing the controls for different materials.

Matching the LVA to the individual child

These should be prescribed by an appropriately trained person at a Low Vision Unit. Different magnifications may be needed for different tasks. The approximate magnification necessary is worked out by comparing the size of the task detail to the person's comfortable print size (not their near acuity, which is the smallest print they can see, but which will be read slowly and with difficulty).

eg   Child's comfortable print size = N36
        Size of print to be read = N12
        Magnification = 3x

If the size of print to be read was N6, the magnification needed by the same child would be 6x.

Other factors need to be taken into consideration when deciding on the type of LVA and level of magnification. Children's visual impairment may mean that certain LVAs are unsuitable for them. As a rule children with impaired visual acuity benefit most from optical LVAs whereas for instance, a child with retinitis pigmentosa and tunnel vision, but normal visual acuity would probably not benefit from them. Children need huge encouragement to see the benefit of LVAs and overcome feeling self-conscious about using something different from their sighted peers. In particular LVAs given them greater access to written material which has not been specifically modified for them. Being able to look at CD covers, magazines and cereal packets promotions may be more motivating than being able to read a textbook!

TRAINING IN THE USE OF FUNCTIONAL VISION

It has increasingly become accepted that it is important to encourage and train children to use their vision to the full, whilst providing them with the optimal environment, materials and technology. This involves:

i)   learning to use the other senses
ii)   training in the efficient use of functional vision

i)   *Learning to use the other senses*
        If children have impaired vision they, to a greater or lesser
        degree, rely on their other senses. The most obvious one is
        hearing. Sight has various degrees of usage; the glancing
        'seeing' which takes in the general picture but doesn't pick out
        details, is different to concentrated *'looking'* where the viewer
        is working hard and using sight to gain specific information. In
        the same way, hearing can have various degrees of attention.
        Seeing could be equated with hearing, and looking with
        listening. Visually impaired children will not automatically listen
        with concentration, nor be able to interpret and use different
        sounds. In order for them to become skilled at listening, the
        following should be part of the visual impairment education
        programme.

        a) Learning to use equipment
           Tapes can be a significant tool in a visually impaired
           children's education, especially as they get older and have
           to cope with increasingly large amounts of information. It
           is important, then, that the child is familiar with the
           controls of a tape recorder, so that using tapes helps rather
           than hinders. The facility of variable speed on some tape
           recorders means it is possible to listen to speech at a speed
           of around 250 words per minute, which is about the same
           as a good silent print-reading speed; spoken speech is
           usually about 100 words per minute. Another important
           feature is tone-indexing, which allows the listener to find a
           specific section on a tape quickly, without having to listen
           to the whole tape. It works by using different tones to
           mark parts of the text eg three short tones could indicate
           the start of a chapter. Once familiar with the meaning of
           the tones, the child can move quickly about the tape.

b) <u>Listening skills</u>
The child needs to be able to listen for:
- factual details
- the main point of the passage
- whether opinion or fact is being presented

When young, children can play listening games eg recognising familiar sounds, picking out one sound from background noises etc. As they get older, children need to be questioned by the carer. This can be done in conjunction with training for speed listening. The carer could give the child a passage to listen to for the main points, set at a speed which is the maximum that is comfortable. With practice, it should be possible to increase the speed gradually.

c) <u>Interpreting the sound environment</u>
Visually impaired children should also be taught to interpret sounds in the environment. This will help their understanding of the world in which they live and move, and aid orientation and mobility. So although we have said it is valuable to have a learning environment in which background noises are muffled, it would not be good if all such noises were cut out altogether. Many noises give clues as to what is going on. For example the sound of doors opening and closing may alert a child to the entrance or exit of a person to the room. The sound of chalk on a blackboard can be recognized as a signal that significant notes are being made, and can be a cue for a blind child to start noting the teacher's speech straight away, without:

- needing to be told to take notes, or
- missing the vital first sentences.

The ability of a visually impaired child to move around familiar and unfamiliar places can be increased through organized mobility training that includes:

- The recognition of common sounds such as clocks, office sounds. The location of certain fixed sounds, such as a clock above the doorway, can be memorised and used to help visually impaired children move around with more confidence.

- The use of reflected sound. Studies have shown that it is possible to become aware of an object in one's path by hearing reflected sound coming back from that object. Echo-detection or echo-location means using this phenomenon by actively listening to returning sound, or even deliberately making noises in order to interpret the echoes made. Such deliberate noises could be tongue snapping, finger clicking or stamping. In one study, blind people making artificial noises were able to distinguish a disc covered in velvet from one covered in denim. Knowing how different objects sound give clues as to when there is an absence of an object such as a doorway, or an open door. The obvious drawback to making deliberate noises is that it draws attention to the visually impaired person. Nevertheless, it could be one strategy that some children find useful. Training in this is part of mobility specialists' expertise, and advice in training programmes should be sought from them.

ii) *Training in the efficient use of functional vision*
In the earlier part of the 20th century there was a tradition in European schools for blind children that visually impaired children should not be encouraged to use their eyes, in order to prevent further deterioration of vision. This was the medical view, and so was largely supported by the educationalists. There was also a tendency to classify most visually impaired children as blind, and thus to treat them as having no useful vision at all. These views began to change in the mid 1900s. Dr Natalie Barraga from the University of Austin, Texas, USA, was one of the first educationalists to act on the changing medical views. Ophthalmologists began to believe that the practice of *'sight-saving'* by not using their eyes at all had no

medical justification in most cases; furthermore, the work of psychologists was finding that lack of visual stimulation could lead to a lessening of visual functioning, whereas specific training could lead to improvements in discrimination. Dr Barraga's work in the 1960s showed that children classified as blind could be taught to perceive and manage their near environment using their functional vision as well as their other senses. This has great implications for visual impairment education in the developed world, as the majority of visually impaired children have some potentially useful vision. Her work was the basis for a British project based at the University of Birmingham, which produced a handbook for teachers, 'Look and Think', whose aim was the visual perception training of visually impaired children aged 5-11. It provides a useful checklist of the skills involved in visual perception; a means of assessing whether an individual possesses those skills, and most importantly, suggestions for training the child in those specific skills, so that a less developed skill can become fully developed. These areas of visual perception include:

- depth perception
- 3D discrimination
- perspective
- line drawings
- photos
- facial expressions and body language
- patterns and symmetry

In order for visually impaired children to begin to use their vision most efficiently, they must be encouraged to look properly; to be trained in scanning and search procedures. They should find such training interesting and rewarding, for they might well be too accustomed to not seeing and therefore feel no incentive to look for visual information. Training in these skills should be part of an overall programme of learning to use functional vision which includes all the points made in this chapter. Rather than be a tick-list of skills to be covered, training visually impaired children to use their functional vision should be tailored to their individual needs, and involve a lot of creative common sense. Observe the child and identify strengths and weaknesses, then work out what can be done to overcome any problems that exist. Above all, remember that the child will be in school, with all its support systems, for only a few years, and the ultimate objective of any training programme should be to enable the visually impaired child to cope as well as possible in a world that still makes few allowances for visual impairment. Newspapers will not necessarily be enlarged for her, obstacles on the pavement may not be removed, and a good training programme will have provided the young person with the strategies and confidence to deal with such challenges.

Continuing visual assessment on a day-to-day basis
Normally, the first assessment of a visually impaired child will have been carried out by the doctors who diagnosed the visual impairment. It will have included the assessment of near and distance vision, but significantly, the tests will have been carried out in clinical conditions. It is important, therefore, that visually impaired children are assessed by teachers of the visually impaired for near and distance vision as described in this chapter, and that any information gathered is conveyed to others. As stressed before, the visual acuity and print size should be one that the child finds comfortable in normal surroundings, rather than the absolute best that can be seen, which is hard to sustain during a whole lesson.

However, once an initial assessment has been carried out, it is important that there are regular formal and informal assessments throughout the child's education by teachers of visually impaired children. How often the formal assessment is carried out will depend on the resources of the staff; once a term is probably a good target.

The formal assessment should include:
- The near and distance acuity of the child. Once print size has been determined, one idea is to time how long the child takes to read quite a long passage in classroom

conditions, and to repeat the exercise termly, to check whether the print size is still comfortable. If it becomes clear that the child is taking longer to read a similar passage, then print size needs to be reassessed. If the child reads aloud, it might also be possible to determine whether the child is struggling in other areas, such as finding the next line, going back to search for information, scanning text to get an overview. These are all study skills which are important for learning and may need to be taught. For distance acuity, find an empty classroom and write on the blackboard or whiteboard. See if the child can still see the same size writing from the same distance. If not, the child or teacher of visually impaired children should ask for class seating arrangements to change.

- Checking that the chosen print size is comfortable in all media used eg novels, maths books, computer screens. Remember that an intermediate acuity might be required for reading music, or public reading.
- Testing peripheral vision as explained in Chapter 2.
- Testing colour vision. This can be done using commercial tests such as Ishihara, or by simply asking the child about coloured objects spaced around the room, or illustrated in books. Special attention needs to be given to the background contrast.
- Checking the child's lighting and seating requirements are still the same.
- Checking that the child is comfortable with any technology and LVAs. Regular speed tests with the child's technology such as laptops, and his or her LVAs can show if they are being used successfully.
- Regular liaison with the class teachers involved with the visually impaired child, to anticipate and deal with any issues before they become problems. A simple, quick to use tick-sheet can be used, and if any problems are identified, then teachers of the visually impaired can spend time solving them, and giving support where it is needed.

There is also scope for informal assessment. Observation of how visually impaired children move around school is very helpful, as is classroom observation. Is the LVA being used appropriately? Is the child joining in class and group activities or is it clear that some support is necessary? Is the child able to ask for better lighting or seating? Is there any imagery in the worksheets which is not seen or misinterpreted because it is too small or of the wrong contrast? Such observations will help the teacher of the visually impaired plan an appropriate programme for each child.

<u>Working to the same agenda as the family</u>
The relationship between the carer of the visually impaired child and teaching staff is very important. Good communication between home and school means that useful information is pooled and available to all those involved with visually impaired children, so that problems at home or school can be solved before they begin to hinder progress. If teachers and carers agree on using common vocabulary and strategies, visually impaired children can only benefit from the constant reinforcement and encouragement. It is particularly important with younger children or visually impaired children with additional learning difficulties that school and home use the same vocabulary to avoid confusion and aid reinforcement.

Carers of visually impaired children are clearly the best people to give teaching staff information on the day-to-day implications of a child's visual impairment. They are the ones who will have noticed certain habits or problems or abilities the child has. They can give suggestions as to what may motivate the child and what interests may be used to help in his or her education. They are also able to inform staff about any relevant medical information. Of course it is also crucial to involve the child in all of this too - it is the child who should lead the way.

The flow of information should be two-way. It is important that teachers ensure that carers are informed about what is going on at school. Clearly, the education of visually impaired children is best carried out as a team effort, with input from all those involved. How such consultation takes place, whether it be formally or informally, is down to the individuals concerned, but staff should ensure that communication with the child's carers remains a priority. A diary which *'belongs'* to the child and is filled in by all interested parties can prove very helpful.

APPENDIX A

GLOSSARY OF TERMS

Accommodation   The name given to the shape change of the lens, (which becomes thicker and rounder) to allow focusing on near objects. This flexibility is lost with age (presbyopia). The average age of presbyopia is 45 years, when reading glasses are usually required.

Agnosia   Disorder of processing sensory information. There are many different types and agnosia forms a suffix for words such as 'prosopagnosia' and 'simultanagnosia'.

Akinetopsia   This is a condition in which there is an inability or difficulty in seeing moving objects. This is associated with damage on both sides of the brain, just in front of the area responsible for vision. In this condition, children and adults are able to see and analyse material that does not move. However when it does move it is less easily seen. The quicker an object is moving the harder it becomes to see it, until fast moving objects are no longer seen at all.

Albinism   Genetic disorder involving lack of pigment (colour) in the eyes and/or skin.

Amblyopia   This is a type of visual impairment resulting from inadequate development of the visual pathways during young childhood. It may occur when images formed by an eye are degraded during the early years of life due to for example, uncorrected refractive error, or untreated cataract or corneal opacity. This is called deprivational amblyopia. It can also occur if one eye is squinting and the brain suppresses the vision from it to avoid double vision (strabismic amblyopia).

Aniridia	Genetic disorder in which the iris is almost completely absent.
Antibodies	Proteins produced in the blood to fight infections. They can be measured by looking at a blood sample in the laboratory and may therefore help to diagnose the presence of a particular infection such as rubella or toxoplasma.
Aphakia	Absence of the lens of the eye, usually due to surgical removal of a cataract. This condition produces marked long-sightedness and requires thick spectacles, contact lenses or a surgically implanted intraocular lens to correct it.
Aqueous humour	Transparent fluid which fills the front of the eye, giving the eye its pressure (which is called intraocular pressure).
Astigmatism	Sometimes illustrated by considering the front of the eye to be shaped like a rugby ball rather than a football (as it should be). The curvature and hence the focusing power of the eye is different in different directions. This is corrected by using cylindrical optical lenses (spectacle or contact) instead of spherical.
Blindsight	This is a condition in which there is absent vision at a conscious level due to damage to the visual cortex. However, such children may be able to see to walk about without bumping into anything, and may well have fairly good vision for moving targets. This vision is primarily to the side and probably does not involve central vision. It may be due to intact visual function in the part of the brain responsible for perception of movement, which is absent in those people with akinetopsia.
Buphthalmos	From the Greek meaning 'Ox-eye' - glaucoma in children's eyes can produce enlargement of the eyes because of their elastic walls.

Cataract	The name given to loss of transparency of the lens. Commonly age-related but can also be due to trauma, or can be present from birth (congenital). It is the commonest cause of blindness worldwide, (adults and children) preventable if enough surgery were carried out.
Choroid	Coloured layer behind the retina at the back of the eye containing many blood vessels.
Ciliary body	The pump which supplies aqueous humour to the eye (making it from blood).
Cognitive visual disorders	These usually result from damage to parts of the visual cortex and may involve specific problems such as inability to recognise faces or difficulty in simultaneously processing multiple pieces of visual information.
Colour blindness	This is usually used to describe genetically inherited anomalies of cone receptors which would better be termed 'colour confusion'. Such conditions do not have significant educational implications. Some visually impaired children such as those with cone dystrophies, optic nerve disease or cortical visual impairment, may have abnormal or reduced colour perception.
Cone cells	The less numerous photoreceptors used for central, detailed vision and colour vision.
Congenital	Any condition with which a child is born.
Contrast sensitivity	The ability to distinguish different shades of grey from each other - an important aspect of functional vision. Formal assessments such as the Peli Robson chart are available. Colour contrast sensitivity entails the ability to distinguish varying shades of colour, for example a light blue from a darker blue.

Cornea	The transparent front surface of the eye which covers the coloured part and focuses incoming light.
Corneal graft	An operation in which a scarred or damaged cornea which has lost its transparency is replaced by a 'donor' cornea removed from someone who has died recently. Very fine nylon thread is used to suture the new cornea into place. There is a risk of rejection and many hospital follow-up visits are required in the first two years after the operation.
Crowding	A phenomenon seen in disorders of the visual brain such as amblyopia or cortical visual impairment. If too much visual information is presented to the child at once then visual performance is reduced, whereas good responses may occur when one target is presented at a time.
Emmetropia	Normal ocular optics: that is, no correcting lens is necessary to produce optimum vision from the eye. Visual impairment may or may not be present.
ERG	Stands for electroretinography, a method of assessing vision in children unable to co-operate with subjective methods and also helpful for making diagnoses such as retinitis pigmentosa. The technique involves measuring the electrical signals generated in the retina in response to visual targets.
Fovea	Centre of macula (2mm across), where the cones are densely packed. The fovea is the most important point in the retina for detailed vision.
Functional vision	The ability to use eyesight in everyday conditions.

Genetic inheritance A condition passed on from generation to generation through an abnormality in the genes. Some people may have the abnormal gene without having the disease (carrier). There are four main types of such inheritance:

Autosomal dominant inheritance
We all have two copies of each gene. In these conditions only one of the copies has to be abnormal for the disease to occur so the disease may be passed on from just one parent. As a result, a family tree may show several affected generations. In general when there is such a family history, there will be an approximately 50% chance of any child of the affected parent inheriting the disease. The number of affected or unaffected children already born to the parent does not affect the risk to any future children; it will always be roughly 50%.

Autosomal recessive inheritance
In these conditions, both copies of the gene have to be abnormal (one normal copy of the gene is sufficient to protect against the disease) and therefore the disease has to be inherited from both parents. The diseases therefore tend to be rarer because they depend on the coincidental reproduction from two unaffected carriers (without the disease because each has only one gene affected) The parents will therefore not know that they are both coincidentally carriers of the disease until their first affected child is born. Any child born to such parents has a one in four chance of being affected and unaffected children have a 67% chance of being carriers. Family trees with affected patients in multiple generations are uncommon in recessive conditions.

Sex-linked recessive
In these conditions, the gene abnormality is carried on one of the sex chromosomes (a chromosome is a strand of genetic material) called the X chromosome. Females have two of these whereas males have one X and one Y chromosome. As for other recessive conditions (see above), one normal copy of the gene is sufficient to protect against it and therefore in general, females do not have the disease because it is very unusual for both their X chromosomes to be affected, but males do get the disease because there is no 'spare' normal X chromosome to protect against it. Females with the abnormality in one of their X chromosomes are therefore unaffected carriers for the disease and their sons will have a 50% chance of having the disease and their daughters will have a 50% chance of being carriers.

Maternal inheritance
An unusual inheritance pattern, where both sexes can be affected by the disease but only the mother can pass it on to her children for example with Leber's optic neuropathy.

Glaucoma	Group of eye disorders relating to raised pressure inside the eye.
Homonymous hemianopia	This literally means 'same-sided half-blindness'. A left homonymous hemianopia means that the left half of vision from both eyes is absent and that a person can only see things on the right side. It can be produced in a variety of conditions affecting the visual brain and pathways after they have crossed at the optic chiasm.
Hypermetropia (hyperopia)	Long sightedness. Things seen more clearly in the distance than at near.

Iris	The coloured part of the eye which is also joined to other coloured parts of the eye, the ciliary body and the choroid, which are not visible without special instruments. Together they make up the uvea. Because the iris is coloured, light cannot pass through it, but instead must pass through the central hole in the iris called the pupil.
Ishihara test	A test for colour confusion.
Lens	Transparent structure (similar in shape to a Smartie) situated behind the pupil. Flexible shape allows variable focusing (accommodation) in young people. Loss of transparency is called cataract.
Low Vision Aids (LVAs)	The term can apply to anything that improves a person's functional vision, but is normally used when referring to optical LVAs, that is, those that use lenses. Examples include hand-held magnifiers and Closed Circuit TVs (CCTVs).
Maclure Reading Test	A standard reading card designed to measure near vision.
Macula	Central (4mm across) area of the retina which contains most of the cones and is responsible for central and colour vision (it includes the fovea).
Myopia	Short sightedness. Things seen more clearly when near than when in the distance.
Nystagmus	Unstable or 'wobbly' eyes. Usually due to certain types of visual impairment eg cataract, albinism or cone dystrophy, but sometimes due to abnormalities in the parts of the brain which control eye movement such as the cerebellum.
Ophthalmologist	A doctor who has special qualifications and experience with disorders of the eye and treating them with appropriate medicine and surgery. Also known as eye doctors or eye surgeons.

Ophthalmoscope	A special instrument used by optometrists and ophthalmologists to view the retina. It consists of a torch and lens combination.
Optic chiasm	The (partial) crossover of the optic nerves whereby behind the crossover, all signals from the left side of our vision (of both eyes) are processed in the right side of the brain and vice versa.
Optic disc	The exit point of the optic nerve from the eye, seen with an ophthalmoscope, and susceptible to damage in glaucoma.
Optic nerves	The nerves which carry visual signals from the retina to the brain. They cross over in part at the optic chiasm.
Optometrist	A person who specialises in measuring and prescribing corrections for refractive errors. Also known as ophthalmic opticians, they may work in a high street shop or a hospital department or both. They are also trained to screen for common medical and surgical problems of the eye such as glaucoma and cataract.
Orthoptist	A person who specialises in assessing certain aspects of children's vision, usually with a particular interest in the management of squint and amblyopia.
Paediatrician	Doctor who specialises in child health.
Peripheral vision	Although our detailed vision is confined to the thing we are looking at any given time, we are also aware of shapes and movements in the edge of our vision. This is very important in our awareness of where we are in space and in helping us to move about.
Photoreceptors	Rod and cone cells in the retina which convert light energy into electrical nerve signals to the brain.

Phthisis	Collapse of the eye due to failure of production of aqueous humour – indicates serious damage to the eye, which will be blind.
Presbyopia	The normal loss of accommodation which is seen with age.
Prosopagnosia	This is a condition in which there is a disability in recognising faces. It is particularly associated with left hemianopia, as it is related to problems of the right visual cortex. In order to recognise people we have to have a store of faces in our minds. If we are unable to build up or access such a store, then the ability to recognise faces is impaired.
Pupil	The hole (aperture) in the iris which appears as a black circle in a normal eye. The size alters according to the amount of light shining on the eye to regulate how much light enters the eye and to increase depth of focus.
Refraction	This is the process by which the eyes are measured for long or short sightedness and/or astigmatism.
Refractive error (emmetropia)	The absence of emmetropia that is, the presence of hypermetropia, myopia or astigmatism or any combination thereof. Visual impairment may or may not be present.
Retina	The screen of the eye onto which the picture is projected (like the film of a camera). It is made up of rods, cones and nerve cells which link to the visual brain.
Retinoscopy	An objective method of refraction suitable for use with babies or those with learning difficulties. It is performed by ophthalmologists and optometrists.
Rod cells	The more numerous photoreceptors used for peripheral vision and for low illumination levels.

Sclera	The white of the eye; a strong coat for the eyeball to protect the delicate structures within.
Scotoma	An area of the visual field where visual sensitivity is reduced (relative scotoma) or completely absent (absolute scotoma).
Simultanagnosia	This is a condition in which complex pictures cannot be simultaneously processed. This most commonly occurs in children who have quadriplegia and who have damage to both sides of the brain in the central region. Such children may only be able to access part of a picture. For example, they may look at a picture of a bicycle and say they see a wheel, but are unable to see the picture as a whole. One strategy for the management of this condition is to build up pictures sequentially using simple, large images one at a time.
Snellen chart	The most common method of testing visual acuity. It consists of black letters of different sizes on a white background, held at six metres from the person being tested. The smallest letter that can be read is taken as a measure of acuity and the result is expressed as a fraction eg six over sixty, which indicates that an eye can read at six metres away what a normal eye could read at sixty metres away.
Strabismus (squint)	Failure of alignment of the two eyes, such that they are looking at two different objects simultaneously instead of at one. Often in children the second image is suppressed by the brain so that they do not see double.
Topographic agnosia	This condition is a disability in route finding, both on large and a small scale, and commonly accompanies prosopagnosia.

Uvea	The iris, ciliary body and choroid together make up the uvea.
VEP	Stands for 'visual evoked potential', an electrical technique for assessing vision, measuring electrical signals generated in the visual cortex.
Visual acuity	A measure of the finest detail that can be seen by an eye under optimum conditions.
Visual cortex	The cortex refers to parts of the surface areas of brain responsible for conscious perceptions, thoughts and actions. The visual cortex consists of a primary visual (striate) cortex which receives the signals directly from the eyes and secondary (visual association) areas responsible for various aspects of complex analysis of vision such as shape or face recognition or detection of movement.
Visual field	This is simply everything that can be seen by an eye in any one position, and includes the detailed central vision as well as the peripheral vision.
Vitreous gel	Transparent gel filling the back of the eye.

APPENDIX B

BLINDNESS AND VISUAL IMPAIRMENT DEFINITIONS

World Health Organization guidelines for classifying levels of vision in childhood are based on three types of measurement:

1   **Distance visual acuity (with both eyes open)**
- Visual impairment – visual acuity less than 6/18 but better than or equal to 6/60.
- Severe visual impairment – visual acuity of less the 6/60 but better or equal to 3/60.
- Blind – visual acuity of less than 3/60.

2   **Functional vision**
- Can see to walk around. Tested by getting the child to walk between two chairs, placed 1 metre apart.
- Can recognise faces. The child is able to identify a person known to them by visual recognition of face alone at a distance of 3 metres.
- Can see print. A cross, square or circle about 2 cm in size is drawn and the child is asked to describe or copy it.
- Believed to have useful residual vision (where formal testing not possible).
- Defined as sufficient vision for at least one of the following:
  - independent mobility
  - making social contacts
  - near vision

3   **Visual fields**
Some assessment of visual field should be made for all children, though categories are not specified for this (see Chapter 2).

This classification is designed to be possible to perform in any situation, in any country, however limited facilities are. It recognises that visual acuity is not the only measure of visual function. Some children will have an acuity of poorer than 6/18 for distance but still function remarkably well educationally, whereas others with acuities better than 6/18 may have significant impairment of visual function due to cognitive dysfunction or gross field deficits. In practice the best definition for visual impairment in children is any impairment of visual function sufficient to require special educational assistance.

APPENDIX C

COMMON MYTHS

1   Sitting close to the television can harm your eyes

There is no evidence that sitting close to a TV causes any harm to the eyes. It is just considered antisocial because it blocks the view for others. Children with visual impairment choose to sit at the distance they can see the pictures, so by telling them to sit back from the TV you are impairing their enjoyment and education because they can't see the programme any more!

2   Children should be barred from activities because of poor vision

Automatic bars on children's activities because they might hurt themselves probably do more harm than good because educational opportunities are lost. With appropriate support most children with impaired vision can and do take part in a wide range of sports and physical activities. If there are safety concerns, appropriate assessment under supervision will allow any risks to be addressed in a positive manner.

3   The assistant should escort and look after the child

Children included in mainstream education often have an adult who escorts them to school. A learning support or teaching assistant may also accompany them to varying degrees in the day. It is a difficult balancing act to ensure that the assistant's presence aids rather than impairs social inclusion and the development of mobility. It is essential that assistants receive training for this important role.

4 You can strain your eyes

Eyes are unstrainable! It doesn't matter how close reading material is, or how long you read for, the eyes cannot be harmed.

5 VDUs harm your eyes

They don't! There is no scientific evidence showing that VDUs and computer screens can harm the eyes. They may cause headaches but they do not cause eye damage.

BIBLIOGRAPHY

- 'Show me what my friends can see'
  Patricia Sonksen & Blanche Stiff, Institute of Child Health,
  London, 1991

- 'Teaching children with visual impairments'
  Anthony B Best, Open University Press, 1995

- 'The visually handicapped child in your classroom'
  E K Chapman & J M Stone, Cassell, London, 1988

- 'Assessment of vision in children'
  L Hyvarinen, Fack, Sweden, Tomteboda School, 1983

- 'Foundations of education for blind and visually handicapped
  children and youth: theory and practice'
  G T Scholl, New York, American Foundation for the Blind, 1986

- 'Look and think handbook and teacher's file'
  M J Tobin & E K Chapman, Schools Council, London and
  Royal National Institute for the Blind, 1989

- 'Blindness and early childhood development'
  D H Warren, New York, American Foundation for the Blind,
  1984

- 'Paediatric opththalmology'
  David Taylor, Blackwell Science, Second edition, 1997

- 'The management of visual impairment in childhood'
  Alistair R Fielder, Anthony B Best and Martin C O Bax, Clinics in
  developmental medicine No.128, Cambridge University Press,
  1993

- 'Childhood blindness: a new form of recording visual loss in
  children'
  C Gilbert, A Foster, A-D Negrel and B Thylefors, Bulletin of the
  World Health Organization 71 (5): 485-489, 1993

RECOMMENDED READING

- 'AFB practice report: show me how'
  M Brennan, American Foundation for the Blind, 1982

- 'Building blocks: foundations for learning for young blind and visually impaired children'
  B Dominguez and J Dominguez, American Foundation for the Blind, 1991

- 'Can't your child see?'
  J and S Freeman, Pro.ed Publications, 1995

- 'The world in our hands' (set of five videos and booklets for parents of visually impaired children)
  Royal National Institute for the Blind, 1993

- 'Children with visual impairments in mainstream settings - a guide for teachers'
  Christine Arter, Heather L Mason, Steve McCall, Mike McLinden, Juliet Stone, David Fulton Publishers, 1999

- 'One of the class' (folder for all those involved in the education of visually impaired pupils in mainstream secondary schools)
  Royal National Institute for the Blind, 2000

- 'Towards excellence - effective education for students with visual impairments'
  Pat Keeley and Gillian Gale, Royal Institute for Deaf and Blind Children, Australia, 1998

- 'A vision shared' (video which promotes and identifies aspects of good practices and strategies for the successful inclusion of visually impaired children and young people into mainstream education) Royal National Institute for the Blind, 1999

The above can be ordered via the RNIB Book Sales Service c/o Customer Services Centre, PO Box, 173, Peterborough PE2 6WS
Tel: 0845 7023153 Fax: 01733 371555 Email: cservices@rnib.org.uk
Website: www.rnib.org.uk

INDEX

Abetalipoproteinaemia 96
Accommodation 10,11
Achromatopsia 91
Aids (HIV) 67,68
Albinism 73
Amblyopia 28,35
Aniridia 12,75
Aphakia 64
Aqueous humour 11
Astigmatism 37

Batten's disease 102
Behr's disease 107
Best's disease 99
Blind spot 47,48
Buphthalmos 11,76

Cardiff cards 41
Cataract 8,10,63
Central vision 12,14
Cerebral palsy 45,89,114
Choroid 16,67
Ciliary muscle 9
Closed circuit TVs (CCTVs) 131,136
Cockayne's syndrome 97
Coloboma 71
Colour confusion 24,130
Colour contrast 22,51,53
Cone dystrophy 92
Cones 12,13
Congenital heriditary 61
endothelial dystrophy (CHED)
Congenital hereditary 61
stromal dystrophy (CHSD)
Conjunctiva 57,58
Contrast sensitivity 51

Convergent squint 37
Cornea 9,11,55
Corneal dystrophies 60
Corneal grafting 58,59
Cortical visual impairment 108
Cryptophthalmos 69
Cytomegalovirus (CMV) 67

Diabetes 104,107
DIDMOAD syndrome 106
Down's syndrome 59,60,64

Electroretinogram (ERG) 51

Fovea 12,14,15
Friedreich's ataxia 107
Fundus albipunctatus 91

Glaucoma 11,16,76

Hemianopia 17,31,49
Homonymous 49,50
Hydrocephalus 116
Hypermetropia 34,35

Incontinentia pigmenti 101
Iris 12

Joubert's syndrome 98
Juvenile retinoschisis 100

Kearns-Sayre syndrome 97
Keratoconus 59
Keratoglobus 60

Leber's amaurosis 93
Leber's optic neuropathy 105
Lens 9
Leucodystrophy 103

Low vision aids (LVAs)   32,131

Maclure charts   44
Macular disorders   24,32,125
Macular oedema   95,96,98
Magnifiers   132,134
Metabolic diseases   62
Microphthalmos   67-72
Mucopolysaccharidoses   98
Myopia   34,35,77

Near acuity   43,44
Nerve fibres   106,107
Nieman-Pick disease   103
Norrie's disease   101
Nystagmus   31,43

Oguchi's disease   91
Optic atrophy   67, 106
Optic chiasm   17,49,107
Optic disc   12,16
Optic nerve   12,13,16,17
Optic nerve hypoplasia   104
Optic tracts   17
Optical iredectomy   56

Peripheral vision   14,31
Peter's anomaly   55
Photopigments   12,14
Photoreceptors   12,47
Pigmentary retinopathy   67
Posterior polymorphous   61
dystrophy (PPMD)
Prosopagnosia   113
Pupil   12,35

Refraction   33
Refsum's disease   96,98
Reiger's anomaly   77

Retina   2
Retinitis pigmentosa   95
Retinopathy of prematurity   88
Retinoscopy   34,35
Retrolental fibroplasia   88
Rods   12,52,90
Rubella   59,64,67,68

Sclera   9
Sclerocornea   55
Scotoma   48
Septo-optic dysplasia   104
Snellen chart   38-43
Stargardt's disease   99
Stationary cone disorders   91
Stationary night blindness   91,94
Syphilis   67,68

Tay Sachs disease   103
Toxoplasma   67,68,69

Usher's syndrome   73,96
Uvea   16
Uveitis   77

Visual acuity   15,32,39
Visual cortex   17,19
Visual evoked potential (VEP)   53
Visual field   15,49
Vitamin A deficiency   59
Vitreous   12

Xerophthalmia   59